Listen To Your Body

❧

And Add 10-15 Happy Healthy Years To Your Life

To Victor.
Best Wishes
Lyle Becker

Lyle Becker

Caliana Publishing Co.

Caliana Publishing Co.
328 Northridge Road
Santa Barbara, CA 93105

Content: 1) Physical Health
             2) Mental Health
             3) Happiness

Library of Congress Catalog Number: 99-098131

ISBN No. 0-9661143-1-0

DEDICATION

To my wife Dolores and our eight children
all of whom I love dearly.

THANKS

To writing instructors Richard O'Connor and Cork Milner of
Santa Barbara City College, my editor Nancy Marriott, and my
son Jonathan Becker who designed the cover and did the prepress
work for the book.

ALL PROFITS

From this book will be donated to the Caliana Foundation to help the
less fortunate in the world, in loving memories of Callie and Anna, two
very caring women; mothers of Dolores and Lyle Becker.

TABLE OF CONTENTS

TABLE OF CONTENTS
(continued)

IMPORTANT
AUTHOR'S NOTE TO THE READER

The material included herein is intended to complement, not replace the advice of your own physician, psychotherapist or other health care professional, whom you should always consult about your circumstances prior to starting or stopping any medication or any other course of treatment, exercise regimen or diet.

Chapter 1
What It Means to Listen to Your Body

When people asked me what my latest book was about, I told them I was writing about how we can learn to listen to our bodies and add ten or fifteen happy, healthy years to our life span.

I was surprised at the reaction I got from some of the older people. "That's great," several of them said, "but only if the added years are *really* happy and healthy ones!"

We all have the desire to live out our expected span of years in a happy and healthy manner. But for many, to suggest adding another ten or fifteen years to that expected life span is a frightening prospect. What if the added years aren't truly healthy ones? If they aren't, then they most likely won't be happy ones either. No one seems to want longevity without a promise of health and happiness in the bargain.

In this book, I'm going to tell you what I have learned through the years to make my life more peaceful, healthy and happy. Hopefully, I can help you to do the same. My intention is not only to help older people live longer and enjoy some extra retirement years, but also to share with younger people what my wife Dolores and I have learned throughout our 55 years of marriage to add years to our own life span. You will find a wealth of ideas in these pages that will add health and happiness as well as years to your life, whether you are still young and working in a job or profession, or are retired like we are.

People who are healthy and happy naturally live longer than those who are not. I am 76 and Dolores is 78. We both *feel*—and, as some people tell us—*look* like we're in our fifties or sixties. We are both in relatively good health and are looking forward to many more happy, healthy years together.

As Dolores says, "It would be nice to live into my nineties, or maybe even hit the 100 mark. But if I do, I want to be sure I have a sound mind so I can know I'm really here!"

Another response I got from people when I talked about the new book I was writing was: "Sounds great, but what does it mean to 'listen to your body?'"

It probably has never occurred to you, but consider for a moment that your mind and body are in a state of constant communication. For example, when you are hungry, your stomach communicates with your mind by sending it a "hunger pain," telling your mind that food is needed. You may then ask: What kind of food do I want? You can actually ask your body this question and get a response.

When eating out at a restaurant and looking at the menu, you can "try on" the different foods that interest you by imagining you have eaten them already, and then see how they feel inside you. Using this approach, you can keep looking at the menu until your body says, "Hey, that's it." By letting your body make the decisions, you will find more enjoyment in the food you eat and the food will digest better because you had an agreement with your body before eating it.

You can listen to your body when you are considering other decisions, as well. Just imagine that you have already made the decision mentally, one way or the other, and then see how your choice feels in your body. If it feels right, it probably is right. That's what I call a *mind-body* decision.

Now there is scientific proof that your mind communicates regularly with the various organs of your body, and *vice versa.*—a phenomenon known as the "mind-body connection."

I learned about this connection a few years ago when I attended a lecture by Dr. Candace Pert, an internationally known brain researcher who has extensively documented how the body and mind communicate with each other. In 1972, Dr. Pert discovered the opiate receptor, which is a mechanism that underlies much of human emotion, and received the acclaim of the scientific community for her discovery. Her book, *The Molecules of Emotion*, (see reference section) tells us that all organs of the body have tiny receptors on their cells to receive information from the brain. The brain also has these receptors, and can receive information from the organs. She describes how through the body's biochemistry, the organs are in constant communication with each other as well as with the brain. Her research proves scientifically that not only do we have a thinking brain, but a thinking body as well.

The mind-body connection can help us to understand much of what we call health and illness. For instance, sometimes the mind is so preoccupied with thoughts and emotions, it can no longer process them and goes on overload. You may experience the overload as a rise in blood pressure, muscular tension, irritability and even depression—all signs that your mind is affecting your physical well-being. You may also experience headaches or migraines, as I have. Fortunately, about thirty years ago I learned to eliminate simple headaches as well as severe migraines from my life with a simple relaxation exercise that utilizes the mind-body connection. You, too, can learn to do this exercise and never have to rely on medication again.

In this book, I will show you how the mind-body connection helps you to listen to your body, and how you can use it to improve and maintain your health and happiness.

You will learn how I came to ease the physical pain that comes from worry—a mental state of dwelling on the worst that can happen in the future. The excessive stress that comes from worrying can cause pain more severe than even the worst of headaches. For example, I remember a time when things looked so bad in our business that I was constantly worried about bankruptcy. The mental stress caused my body to develop a piercing pain that felt like a spike was driven through my chest into my back. At the same time, I had a sore mouth from grinding my teeth at night. When I stopped worrying about the problem, all of these painful symptoms disappeared.

I'll show you how to drift off to sleep like a baby, without any medication, even when your body is under so much stress that it won't surrender to sleep although dead tired.

You'll learn about *Focusing* in these pages, a technique Dolores and I learned years ago that utilizes the body's physical discomfort or pain to locate and resolve those negative feelings that may be buried inside us, often out of the range of our mind's awareness.

You will also read about how I have struggled all my life with a poor self-image and feelings of insecurity, and the bold new program I am using to improve my self-image and get over this insecurity. I hope my experience will be of help to others who may be plagued with this same problem. I'll also tell you about my lifelong search for happiness, and what I believe is necessary for success in the pursuit of happiness.

An important part of staying healthy and happy into your later years is making sure you take care of yourself physically. A good physical condition can send a message to the mind that all is well, providing it with peace and happiness. That state of mind, in turn, supports our physical health, once again completing the mind-body connection.

I'll relate the story of how I arrived at a healthy, balanced diet and how that changed my life in so many ways. After 20 years, my body rebelled from not eating certain foods to lower my cholesterol, such as eggs, butter, cheese and most fats. When I went on a balanced diet that again included these and other forbidden foods, as recommended by two eminent endocrinologists (specialists in hormones such a cholesterol and insulin), I managed to get my cholesterol back to a normal range. I will tell you why these same specialists maintain that the low-fat, high-carbohydrate diets in vogue for the last 15 years with people trying to lose weight are instead making these people fat. Then I'll tell you what the balanced diet consisted of that kept me from gaining back the ten pounds I lost five years ago due to a severe bronchial illness.

Furthermore, you'll read about why I haven't caught the flu or a cold in the last five years because of what I learned from a medical expert about my immune system. A balanced diet has kept me completely free from illness, and I remain healthy year-round now, with the exception of a few minor symptoms. Before I went on this diet, I had been catching every cold or flu bug that came around the block. You, too, can have a strengthened immune system when you balance your diet.

We all know how important exercise is to our body, but many of us say we can't find the time for it. In this book, I describe an exercise plan you can do in your home that gives a workout to the upper body as well as the heart and lower body. And it only takes 10—15 minutes a day, without requiring any fancy or expensive exercise equipment.

Finally, it's my hope that this book will help you become more aware of how to listen to your body for the benefit of your physical and mental well-being. If so, those 10—15 years you add to your life will no doubt be happy and healthy ones!

Chapter 2
My Search for Happiness

We are all eager to add those happy years to our lives, and this can mean different things to different people. But one thing I've learned in my life is that happiness doesn't happen automatically. I believe if we want to have happiness in our lives, we must be willing to search for it. So I will begin by sharing with you how I searched for and found happiness, and what that has come to mean for me.

Early Life

I remember very little about my childhood, except that as a child I was very unhappy. As the youngest of twelve children, I can imagine my parents were not too enthusiastic about raising another child after averaging a new baby every two years for 24 years.

I don't remember our household being a happy one when I was growing up. Relationships between family members were difficult. I remember arguments between my mother and father, although I don't know what they were about. I heard arguments my father had with one of my brothers when he caught him smoking at a young age, and later on in life, when he wanted to marry a girl who wasn't Catholic. I lived in fear of my father. He would become angry if we kids didn't do things the way he wanted them done or when he wanted them done. I was a submissive child, afraid to speak up, afraid I wouldn't do things right.

As I mentioned in my previous book, *King of the Gumballs*, I can't remember anything that happened during my early years of school, starting after the first day my mother brought me to the Catholic school across the road from our house. I was frightened of this strange new environment and followed her back home. The school didn't have a kindergarten, and, at five and a half years old, I was too immature to be placed in the first grade. I don't remember if my mother took me back to school that same day. The next memory I have about my school experience is being in the seventh grade. During those first six years, I can't remember any of my teachers, where I sat in my classrooms, or anything else.

Those early school years are completely blocked from my memory, probably because I was scared to death most of the time — both at school and at home. I'd heard stories about the nuns at school beating your hands with a ruler if you misbehaved, which undoubtedly made me as docile and scared in school as I was at home. The only memories I have of being at home the first twelve years of my life are mainly unhappy ones — being admonished by my father for forgetting to turn on the electric bed warmer for him at noon (he had TB and had to rest every afternoon), or for not keeping the box filled with kindling so he could heat the water and the bathroom when he got up in the morning. I don't remember ever being slapped or spanked, so I'm sure I was never physically abused.

I have fond memories of my mother when I was a child. Thank God for that, or I probably would have been a worse "basket case" than I was. However, I don't ever remember sitting on her lap or being hugged by her, although I presume from the love she showed to all of us children, including defending us when my dad scolded, that she was probably affectionate toward me. I don't remember my father ever showing affection toward me as a child, although he may have tried. My sister Anita and I both remember a little rhyme he used to say, "Lyle, Lyle, climb on a pile, 'Nita Treata, chase him up a tree."

I'm sure my father wasn't as bad as I make him out to be. It was undoubtedly my extreme insecurity as a child that colored the way I related to him and made our relationship so difficult. Certainly he had plenty of good reasons to not spend much time with his children when we were young. He had built a very successful cigar manufacturing business employing 30 people to make hand-rolled cigars, only to see it evaporate due to the advent of cigarettes and machine-made cigars after World War I. Then, when I was six years old, his bubble burst completely when the stock market crashed and he lost all the money he had made in the business. We went from being one of the wealthiest families in our little town of Brillion, Wisconsin, to near-poverty, as my father desperately tried to find a way to support himself, my mother and the children who were still living at home. The only reminder of the good old days was our large, stately six-bedroom home.

I sensed that my father was a rather proud man, so

such a setback must have been devastating to him. The older children, gone by this time, were raised in the good times, while the rest of us learned what living in the Great Depression was like. We had enough to eat and were better off than many of the people in our small town, but wearing hand-me-down clothing when I was in high school did nothing to help my self-image.

My fondest memories of childhood are all about times when I was away from home — making mud pies and playing games with a young neighbor girl, later playing "Kick-the-can" and "Annie-Annie-over" with the neighborhood kids. When I was older, I remember playing softball on summer evenings with the gang of kids at the end of our block. These enjoyable activities compensated somewhat for the lack of any happiness I can remember having in our home or at school until I was in seventh grade.

Then my life at school got better. Our teacher in seventh grade, Sister Francis George, befriended me, and I acquired two new friends, Carl and Jim. We three boys became inseparable, going places every day — Jim on his bike and Carl on his, and me riding on the back of one of the bikes.

Life at home was getting better, as well. My father had gone into the wholesale candy and tobacco business, and later into the cigarette vending machine business, in order to make a living for his family. I helped my brothers in the summers when they went out in a truck selling candy and cigarettes to the taverns and grocery stores in the surrounding counties. Later on, I helped them on Saturdays and during summer vacations to fill the cigarette machines on their routes. This helped my self-esteem, as I worked hard and took pride in being able to help my brothers. After school, I worked in the cigar factory placing the cigars (made by the one remaining cigar maker) into cellophane tubes, then packed them into boxes. I earned a quarter a week doing this, which I spent every Saturday night at the indoor roller skating rink where I met and skated with girls from Brillion and the surrounding towns.

During high school, I had a breakthrough. In my junior year I was accepted by the "in crowd," the most popular students in our small class of 40 students. Even though their acceptance gave my self-esteem a big boost, I continued to walk the back streets to school each day, afraid I would run into some of my new acquaintances on Main Street. I was afraid I wouldn't know what to say if I met anyone face to face. In my senior year, I was elected class president and editor of the school yearbook, an indication that I must have been quite popular. In spite of my new status, I still didn't have the security to feel comfortable with people on a one-on-one basis, but at least I was having some fun in life.

After graduation, I went to work for the new owner of my dad's former business. A year later, with one of my co-workers, I began a vending business that I developed into a successful national business, as told in my book, *King of the Gumballs*. Looking back, I can see I was not happy working for someone else in an 8-to 5 job. I wanted to find satisfaction in a business of my own.

The next major event in my life-long search for happiness was getting married to Dolores. We were married while I was in the service in World War II, and it was the happiest event of my life. But in just twelve weeks, that happiness turned to fear and worry for both of us when I was sent overseas with the Infantry, and we had to face the possibility I might not return.

The Spirit of Love

As I look back over these early years, I realize I was constantly searching for some kind of happiness in my life. I believe we all are looking for this. But I was looking for a state of permanent happiness, to be in a happy state of mind even when troubling events interfered in daily life. This was what I was really seeking, even though it seemed as unattainable as the pot of gold at the end of the rainbow.

In my search, I decided that an element of personal happiness must be spiritual happiness, since a conscience not fully at rest is surely an impediment to the state of happiness. I began to take time out and go on yearly spiritual retreats. In the quiet of these retreats, I had an opportunity to look into my relationships with others. I always felt better about myself when I returned, usually after three days, to my everyday life.

One of these retreats changed my life. I attended the *Cursillo* (Spanish for "in colors"), a powerful experience in Christian community living that took place over a three-day weekend. The Cursillo consisted of talks and discussions done in groups of six, with 30 men living together and sleeping on cots in a school gym. The group discussions were primarily about how our human relationships could be made more peaceful and happier at home and in the workplace. It was the greatest spiritual experience of my life. As a result of my experiences that weekend, I had the insight that to live in peace with others was probably the road to living in a permanent state of happiness. Beautiful friendships were made in those three days, teaching me that strong relationships are an important part of happiness. I learned how to bring the spirit of love to everyone I met, including store clerks and waitresses, which helped me develop a positive attitude which I still maintain to this day.

The biggest challenge for me, over the years, has been to live that spirit of love every day with those people who are the closest to me — my wife and family. I realized I was nicer to the people at my office than I was to those at home, especially my wife, Dolores. I would say things to her that would hurt her, things I wouldn't think of saying to someone at my office, because if I did, they'd probably quit. My remarks would sometimes provoke an unkind response from Dolores, and sometimes it happened the other way around.

In our early married years, we divided our roles and responsibilities. I was clearly the controlling one, making most of the decisions that affected the two of us, while Dolores made the decisions involving our eight children. After 15 years of marriage, she realized through our separate sessions with a psychiatrist that I'd been controlling her. According to what her therapist said, I had taken over the control function of her sister, who had controlled her before she got married.

At first, it was difficult for me to give up being the one in control and begin to share the decision-making I had done for so long in our marriage. This imbalance was a subject of controversy between us for many years as Dolores asserted herself and claimed her share of the running of our lives. I realized she had a right to be considered in decisions that involved us both, but I was used to having control in my own business and that made it more difficult to give up some of the control at home.

Meanwhile, I enjoyed the years building our vending machine business, even with its ups and downs of profitable years and barely profitable years. However, as I tell about in another chapter, I was never really relaxed about the business. I constantly lived with a low-grade worry about its continued success. This underlying fear didn't cause me to lose much sleep, but it gave me little peace and was certainly not conducive to happiness.

Relocating

Looking for a geographical location in which Dolores and I could make our home and both be happy constituted a large part of my search for happiness.

Every autumn, I would grow despondent at the prospect of the coming Wisconsin winter. The pleasant spring and summer months were over, and I hated the thought of enduring another cold and cloudy Wisconsin winter. I complained to Dolores every year when the fall began, telling her I wished we could get out of Wisconsin for the winter months. I wasn't happy, and I believed it made me unhappy to live in such unpleasant weather for a good part of each year.

Dolores told me she believed happiness is within ourselves, not outside, and if I wasn't happy living in Wisconsin, a change in climate probably wouldn't be the answer. I had to admit there was some wisdom in her words, as she seemed relatively happy herself.

I couldn't move our company office to another part of the country, because our employees couldn't be expected to move with me. But I persisted in wanting to get away in the winters, and Dolores finally agreed to move to St. Petersburg Beach, Florida for the winter months and place our two youngest children, the only ones still living at home, in a Florida school for several months of the school year. We did this for two winters.

After getting a taste of Florida in the winter, I had no desire to go back to living year round in Wisconsin again. I finally persuaded Dolores to move the family and the furniture to a rented house with a swimming pool in Naples, Florida, where we began our third winter. I would rent a small office and run the sales department of our business out of it. The plan was to stay in Florida during the school year and spend the children's summer vacation months in a cottage we had just built in Door County, Wisconsin. Then we would have the best of both worlds—I thought. But Naples was beastly hot compared to St. Petersburg Beach, and in late August when school started, and again into June when school ended, the weather was unbearable for both of us.

It was at this time that Dolores agreed to make a permanent move to Florida and consider it our home. Her only condition was that we relocate near St. Petersburg, where she and the children had made friends and the children would be able to enroll full-time in the same school they had attended before. Dolores also felt the need to own a house and feel "at home" after three years of nomadic existence. Reluctantly, she agreed to sell our house on the Fox River in Appleton, Wisconsin, which meant a great deal to her.

Dolores was more adaptable than I was. She seemed

happy wherever we lived. She told me that if she were unhappy living in Florida, she would still be easier to live with than I was, if we continued to spend winters in Wisconsin. So we purchased a beautiful five-bedroom brick house on a golf course in St. Petersburg where we lived for the next three years.

The climate in St. Petersburg was cooler than Naples, but it wasn't as cool as it had been in nearby St. Petersburg Beach, the town we first lived in. During our third year, when the air conditioning in our home broke down one Labor Day weekend, and we couldn't get it repaired because of the holiday, we both decided it was too hot to stay in Florida. Dolores had come to hate the hot weather as much as I hated the cold weather. But I hated the cold weather too much to return to Wisconsin, and so we moved to Santa Barbara, California.

Looking back, Dolores must have really loved me an awful lot to go along on all those moves. But we both enjoyed living in Santa Barbara, especially after we had settled into our third house.

"This is it," she said. "Next time you want to move, it will be without me." She was kidding, I think.

We remodeled our cottage in Door County on Lake Michigan in Wisconsin and made it our summer home. With the cooler lake breezes in the summer and Santa Barbara's almost perfect climate the rest of the year, Dolores was happy and I was happier. Now, I could no longer blame the weather for any of my unhappiness.

Working on Myself

After we moved to Santa Barbara, I made an effort to

do something about my insecurity and low self-esteem, even though I felt that low self-esteem doesn't in itself make a person unhappy. But it's truly difficult to be happy if you don't like yourself. For several years, I attended self-esteem classes at the City College Adult Education program whenever I had the time, and just let the information sink in. I think it really helped me to feel better about myself.

Several ideas impressed me in these classes. One was about getting the "shoulds" out of our lives—I *should* do this and I *should* do that. The instructor put it more simply: "Don't *should* on yourself," she'd say. "Do things because you want to do them. Look at the things you think you *should* do and sort out the ones you really want to do. Don't let the *shoulds* run your life." Another idea that sunk in was this: If you feel you need changes in your life, your job, your relationship, your education, the weather (as I did), or whatever, don't just keep talking about it—*do* it. As the instructor put it, "If the car never leaves the curb, it won't ever go anywhere."

I began applying these ideas to my life, and found my happiness increasing as I made choices from what I wanted to do, and then doing it.

Finding Happiness in Retirement

It wasn't until I groomed our second youngest son to take over the business and I retired that I finally came close to having true happiness in my life. It had been a lifelong process for me. I hope it doesn't take that long for you, if you've been unhappy in your life.

The business was in a downturn when my son took over, but in a few years, his fresh ideas revived it, and it began to flourish once again. Finally, I was able to let go of my underlying worries about the business continuing to survive through its many ups and downs. I had worried long enough over the 50 years that I built and ran it.

I've come to believe that fear and worry are the greatest obstacles to finding true and permanent happiness. When we get rid of them—by working on what's causing them—up goes the level of happiness in our lives.

Dr. Allison Mayer-Oakes, a geriatrician, in a recent *Santa Barbara News-Press* article says she advises her clients that the secret for growing old happily is "engagement in life, keeping interested in what's happening around you. A social network is really critical. We're social beings," she says, "we need others, someone you know that cares about you. All you need is one person, but more are better. Friends are good medicine" she states, "It's important to keep meeting new people."

Dolores and I have many friends we care about that we feel also care about us. Dolores enjoys corresponding with our friends and keeping in touch. I really appreciate this as if it were up to me I'm afraid it would be only a yearly Christmas card.

Another very important idea for sustaining happiness, I believe, is to find something you are passionate about in life besides your work or career. It's best if you can start developing one or more of these passions before the retirement years begin. Then there isn't likely to be such a big gap from your life's work to your retirement life, and boredom won't have a chance to set in.

Many people can't wait to retire because they aren't really happy with their life's work, or they can't wait to be able to play all the golf, do all the traveling, or get into all the other hobbies they don't have time for prior to retirement.

When I retired from my business several years ago, I didn't know what I would do to prevent boredom. To keep busy, I decided to write a book. Once I got started, it became a passion with me to learn how to write and then to write the story of Dolores' and my life together, about my building the gum and toy vending machine business and her almost single-handedly raising our eight children.

I took some writing courses in the Adult Education program in Santa Barbara. My instructors gave me encouragement and, within three years, I published my first book. The advice one of my instructors gave me on becoming a successful writer was to put down on paper everything I wouldn't otherwise tell people. And that's what I did. Some of our friends, however, thought it was a little too revealing.

I had never gone to college, other than for nine months during my military service, and had never studied writing in high school, so I needed a lot of help writing my story. Now, each day before I begin to write, I take a few minutes to ask for God's help.

My first book, *King of the Gumballs*, was successful, so I decided to continue writing books. As long as God prompts me with the ideas and inspires me with what to put down on paper, I plan to continue writing.

My other passions are gardening and playing duplicate bridge, a tournament bridge game in which you accumulate master points. Other than that, Dolores and I enjoy traveling together, going to the movies, eating out, watching the news together in the evening over a drink, playing backgammon together, and visiting with our children and grandchildren.

A Loving Relationship

I have come a long way in my search for happiness by eliminating fear and worry, developing peace through my spiritual life, finding the ideal places to live for both Dolores and myself, and discovering things I am passionate about doing, both in my business life and in my retirement. But there was still one unsolved problem that seemed to be holding true happiness out of my reach—a more loving relationship with Dolores. We have both been working on it, now that other responsibilities are not foremost in our life.

Our married years have not all been happy ones, as I wrote about in my first book. We have had some serious disagreements and verbal fights through the years.

One evening recently, Dolores and I were watching one of our favorite programs, "Mad About You." A friend who knows us well has told us he sees Dolores and me in the two main characters (and so do we). As we watched this particular episode, we both began to feel a slight rise in anxiety. I spoke first: "That show it pretty close to home." She knew exactly what I meant.

In the episode, Paul Bachman, a documentary filmmaker, and his wife Jamie, who works in public relations, were picking at each other as Dolores and I sometimes do. Like the Bachmans, Dolores and I have both struggled to be in control and wanted to be "right" for much of our married life.

"I'm glad we are getting over that kind of competitiveness in our lives," I said.

Dolores agreed.

In my first book, I told how Dolores almost single-handedly raised our eight children, while I built a national business of gumball vending machines. People who have read that book say Dolores is a saint, and I have to agree. Today, we both acknowledge that many of those years weren't much fun. We often tolerated each other, but didn't show each other much love and affection.

Over the past few years, since I retired, Dolores and I have been more consciously trying to show our love for each other. I've been trying to be more considerate of her needs and wants, and I notice she is doing the same for me. We are also showing each other more affection. Dolores loves to go to the movies. We now have a Sunday ritual — church, brunch and a movie. At home, I do most of the yard and garden work, and I make our bed each day. Dolores made beds for 50 years, so she really appreciates that. I usually wash the dishes that don't go into the dishwasher, and yes, I do windows.

Dolores shows her love in the wonderful dinners she prepares for me —I usually make my own breakfast and lunch—as well as in the dinner parties she creates for our friends to share with us. She says she enjoys cooking. I tell her often how much I appreciate this. Men get to retire, but women don't ever truly retire, because even if they have help with the housework, there's that evening meal to think about each day. Once in awhile, I surprise her. Recently, she was on jury duty and was tired when she came home. I cooked the dinner, and she appreciated it very much.

Recently, we went through a period of attending funerals for several of our friends and relatives. We have been hearing about other friends developing cancer. We thank God that both of us are in good health. Being around all of these health problems has made us think about the day, hopefully far into the future, when this could happen to one of us. We agreed we need to be even nicer to each other and are now making more of a conscious effort to do so. It seems to be working. I'm sure there will be setbacks, but as long as we both try to be "big on nice" (a phrase I got from an old friend), our love and affection for each other will continue to grow.

Browsing through an old book I had around, I came across the best definition I've ever seen for the word *happiness*: "Happiness is a state of mind in which our thinking is pleasant a good share of the time."

I feel I am about as full of happiness as I can be. Dolores seems to be, too. We are blessed. We wish the same for you.

Chapter 3
A Simple Relaxation Exercise Can Add Years To Your Life

Say Good-bye to Headaches, Even Migraines, — Without Medication

I haven't had to take an aspirin or any other medication to cure a headache in 30 years, ever since I learned a simple relaxation exercise that works for me every time.

Since childhood, I have experienced frequent headaches, even migraines, that used to put me in bed for a couple of days with nausea, severe pain over one eye and blurred vision. Then, when Dolores and I attended a relaxation training session about 30 years ago, we learned a technique to cure headaches. But no one ever mentioned this technique could cure migraines as well. I was pleasantly surprised when it did.

I believe migraines and most other headaches are caused by tension from an overload on the brain. I think it's nature's way of making us slow down and rest our mind.

Now when I feel a tension headache coming on and start to get double vision, or I become nauseous because it's the beginning of a migraine, I do this simple relaxation exercise. It might take only a few minutes for a minor headache to disappear, and as much as a half hour to an hour to stop a migraine. The sooner I'm able to start the exercise after the first symptoms, the less time it takes to recover.

Here's what I do: I try to find a quiet place, if possible, because the exercise is easiest to do when there are few distractions. Once, however, I did it in a noisy departure lounge at the Chicago O'Hare airport, and it worked quite well. The only problem was that I fell asleep and missed my plane. Sometimes you can fall asleep without intending to, but according to my instructor, this is not a problem. The body evidently needs the sleep and this is fine—just make sure you're not waiting for a plane.

When I'm at home I find a comfortable upholstered chair or sit on the sofa. I sit up fairly straight, relaxed, and take off my shoes. I let my head drop forward as far as it goes naturally and let my hands relax in my lap. This places a strain on my neck muscles, but I do the exercise so often (for this and other purposes I will tell you about later), that my neck muscles have strengthened, and I no longer get a sore neck.

Then I close my eyes and breathe normally, breathing in and breathing out. I listen to my breathing, being conscious of the air going in and out of my nose and actually hearing the sound I make as I inhale and exhale. When thoughts come into my mind, and I realize I'm listening to them and no longer listening to my breathing, I gently go back to listening to my breathing again. (You can't listen to your breathing and be thinking of something at the same time.) I may have to do this as many as a dozen times during the exercise if my mind is unusually active. I continue until my headache or migraine is completely gone and then go back to whatever I was doing before it began.

That's it. It's such a simple exercise and yet powerful enough to stop the pain of a common headache or severe migraine. (Headaches caused by various sinus conditions may not respond to this relaxation exercise and may need the attention of a doctor.)

Say Good-bye to Insomnia—Without Medication

Another use for this relaxation exercise is to overcome insomnia. If you have trouble getting to sleep at night or waking up and not being able to get back to sleep, doing this exercise can be very effective.

Dolores and I were on an ocean cruise this past year and in order to meet more people, we changed seats at dinner each night. One evening, the conversation was about how to get to sleep at night. One man said he tried the old method of counting sheep, but that didn't seem to work very well. Then a woman at the table said she was having a terrible time getting to sleep, as well as waking up several times during the night and not being able to get back to sleep. She complained that she very seldom had a restful night.

I suggested that she listen to her breathing after she went to bed, and that each time she noticed she was no longer listening to it, to go back gently to doing so. I told her that if she awakened in the night, she should repeat the same process as often as necessary.

The next morning we saw her at breakfast. She said she slept for ten hours, and it was the best night's sleep she'd ever had. She thanked me and gave me a big hug. I was so pleased to have been able to help her.

Once in awhile, when I go to bed at night, I am unusually tense and stiff as a board. In this case, I use another exercise I learned years ago to relax my body before going to sleep. I start at the bottom of my body by wiggling my toes and then letting my toes relax. Then I do the same with my legs, tensing my leg muscles, then letting them relax. Then I do the same with my pelvis, my upper body, my arms and even my face. If I'm not already asleep by the time I reach my head, I use the simple relaxation exercise of listening to my breathing to finish the job.

Because of my age, I usually have to get up to go to the bathroom at night. If I have trouble getting back to sleep, I do the relaxation exercise. If I've already had quite a bit of sleep and don't feel tired, but it's too early to get up, I do the relaxation exercise, and I enter into a kind of twilight sleep. It doesn't feel like I'm really sleeping, but when the alarm goes off I'm always surprised how quickly the time has gone by.

Get Rid of That Tired Feeling

I also use the breathing relaxation exercise during the day if I get sleepy and want to take a catnap to refresh myself.

To do this, I sit up fairly straight but relaxed in a comfortable chair. I let my head drop forward, take off my shoes, sometimes cross my legs, and start listening to my breathing. Again, I return my attention to listening to my breathing every time I find my mind drifting. Can you imagine how happy that brain is to not have all those thoughts bombarding it at one time? I usually go to sleep in five or ten minutes. I may wake up in a half hour, sometimes in an hour or longer. I usually wake up refreshed with no yawning or stretching. I purposely don't lie down on a bed or sofa, because that seems to bring on a different kind of sleep. If I do lie down, I usually have a hard time getting up and tend to roll over and sleep longer. It might be several hours before I get up, and when I do, I yawn and stretch and have a hard time waking up. Also, I find that if I get too much sleep during the day, it can disturb my sleep at night, whereas these shorter catnaps don't interfere with a good night's sleep.

Whenever Dolores and I take a long trip in the car, we usually change off driving. If I'm driving and get sleepy, she takes over the wheel, and I sit in the passenger seat and do the relaxation exercise, waking up a half hour or an hour later, refreshed. Then I go back to driving, and she uses the exercise to get a catnap. We find we can even sleep with the radio on.

Sleeping at home sitting up in a chair with my head bowed down has trained my neck muscles for sleeping in a car, train, or plane, where it's often difficult to tilt the seat back far enough or the seat doesn't go back at all.

Years ago, I used to take frequent plane trips to the Orient on business, often traveling as many as 12 hours without a stop. I found I could eliminate much of my jet lag by sitting up in the plane and using the relaxation exercise to get some sleep. Also, when I arrived at my destination, taking catnaps in a chair when I got tired helped me to function better and get over any remaining jet lag.

When I go to bed at night, I read in bed for ten or fifteen minutes until I get sleepy. I recommend this as a way of becoming tired enough to go to sleep naturally, rather than lying in bed waiting to get tired or having to use the relaxation exercise to sleep. I find this works best for me. But if you need the relaxation exercise to put you to sleep, use it. It can't harm you, and a good night's sleep is important for us all.

Relieve the Stress in Your Life

When you are feeling the effects of stress from daily life, this same simple relaxation exercise of listening to your breathing can help relieve the physical symptoms of stress in your body.

At one time in my life, my body seemed to be continually tense. My arm muscles were always tight, and at night, when I went to bed, my whole body was stiff as a board. When I was finally able to relax and began to fall asleep, my body suddenly jumped, as if jolted by electricity. This jolt, I learned later in a Dale Carnegie course, was not uncommon and often related to stress. Other people in the course had also experienced it during times when they were under great stress.

Using the relaxation exercise, I found a way to eliminate most of the stress in my life that was causing this unpleasant experience at night. When Dolores and I learned the relaxation exercise, I started to use it twice daily to prevent stress from setting in. Shortly after getting up in the morning, I practiced the technique for 15 minutes and then again around 5 PM for the same amount of time. Doing the exercise at the end of the afternoon helped me make the a transition from my office mode to my home and family mode. And since using these twice daily relaxation exercises over the past 30 years, I have rarely felt that disturbing jolt when falling asleep at night.

Also, during the time I was going to work at my office, if I felt tired or stressed, I would close the door, ask people not to bother me or sometimes put up a "Do Not Disturb" sign, and then take 15 or 20 minutes to do my relaxation exercise. I told my employees what I was doing, showed those interested how to do the exercise, and told them they were free to do it at any time they felt the need. Those that didn't have a private office went to the lunch room to do their exercise. It helped me to be more efficient and helped my employees to get over a sleepy feeling or get rid of tension or a headache, or both. This certainly improved their efficiency, too.

Doing this exercise for 15 or 20 minutes twice a day took a lot of discipline when I first started. I wasn't convinced how important it was, and it was easy to put it off. But when I realized I was no longer going around with taut muscles all the time, my entire body seemed to feel better, and this proved the value of doing the exercise to me.

I truly believe that this simple exercise of listening to my breathing has added at least ten years to my life span. After all, walking around all day with tense muscles can't be doing any good for the body. I suggest you add this twice-a-day relaxation exercise to your daily routine, and see for yourself.

Increase Your Creativity

I find that when I'm doing the relaxation exercise, ideas will sometimes pop into my mind. I don't mind this because the ideas are good ones, often about things I haven't thought about before, or things I've wanted to do but had forgotten about. Being in a creative business (as readers know who have read my previous book about my gumball machine business), I needed my mind to be very active.

You've probably had the experience of trying to remember something, and the harder you try, the harder it is to bring that something back into your memory. But at other times, when your mind is relaxed, it's easier to recall something. I believe it's easier to remember something or think of new ideas when your mind is relaxed, rather than racing a mile a minute.

I think this is why I have ideas pop into my mind during my relaxation exercises. Some of my best ideas for building my business came to me while I was using the relaxation exercise, and I can't think of a bad idea or thought that ever came to me while doing the exercise.

I find that writing takes a great deal of concentration and taxes my thought process to the limit. After a few hours, my mind gets tired and sometimes I get sleepy. If I don't stop and use the relaxation exercise to catnap (always sitting upright in a comfortable chair), I get too tired to continue, and therefore am incapable of writing more that day. When I'm sleepy, giving myself a "relaxation-exercise catnap" for a half an hour, an hour, or until I wake up, can refresh me and add several hours to my workday.

When I first learned this simple relaxation exercise, the instructor told us that we would feel more rested from the 15 or 20 minute relaxation exercise, whether we slept or not, than we would if we had slept in bed for several hours. I eventually found this to be true, and as I said before, it doesn't keep you from a good night's sleep. I think the reason for this is because the relaxation exercise primarily rests the mind, which undoubtedly needs some rest during the day. At night, going to bed to sleep rests the mind and the body.

Remember that your body position is very important in the relaxation exercise. Always sit up very straight so you can let your head drop forward. Do not let your head fall back on the upholstered chair or sofa back. If you do, you may fall asleep for hours, getting the kind of sleep you get in bed, resting your body rather than your mind. Also, you may sleep too long with your head back and deprive yourself of a good night's sleep later that night.

I understand Thomas Edison took catnaps in his experimental lab when putting in long days working on his inventions. I like to think that he knew about this relaxation exercise and used it to keep going when he got tired — maybe it even gave him some of his great ideas!

Chapter 4
A New Balanced Diet
Can Control Cholesterol, Weight and Illness

How I Beat My Cholesterol Problem

Five years ago, I had one of the longest and most painful illnesses of my life.

For years, I had been getting colds or the flu several times a year. I don't think I ever passed a winter or spring in my life without becoming ill. If a flu virus came around, I caught it.

Our family doctor convinced me years ago not to rely on antibiotics for these ailments, so I rarely visited him when I was sick. He warned that in the event I might need antibiotics for a serious illness, over-using them could make me immune to their benefits.

But this time, I was sick with symptoms that were worse than any before. My throat was very sore so that whenever I swallowed, which I did often, it felt like I was swallowing ground-up glass. The pain was so severe, I remember thinking that if I had to endure it for the rest of my life, I would certainly pray to die quickly.

Dolores could see the pain I was in and urged me to go to the doctor. When I finally did, he gave me some sulfa pills, which didn't help at all. After a few days of trying the sulfa without relief, I went back to the doctor, and he prescribed antibiotics. Thank God, they worked; I had not become immune to them.

I finally recovered. My illness had lasted almost six weeks. The only consolation I received from the ordeal was losing ten pounds. Before my illness, I was overweight and had been trying to take off the extra pounds. Now, I resolved to keep the weight off that I had lost.

Around the same time as my illness, one of my daughters was seeing Dr. Diana Schwarzbein, a Santa Barbara endocrinologist (a specialist in cholesterol and insulin) because of a hormonal imbalance. She brought back some very interesting literature from her office. I read it all eagerly, and could tell immediately that Dr. Schwarzbein wasn't afraid to stick her neck out in the medical field and break some new ground.

One article, a reprint of a *Santa Barbara News-Press* interview with Dr. Schwarzbein, seemed especially relevant for my own health. I had been unsuccessful in correcting my cholesterol levels, even though I had been on a high-carbohydrate, low-cholesterol, low-fat diet for the previous twenty years. Dr. Schwarzbein was addressing a new way to manage cholesterol levels, a subject well within her specialty field.

In the *News-Press* article, I came across a startling statement by the doctor: "Eating foods high in cholesterol does not increase the blood cholesterol level. Instead, overeating carbohydrates can lead to abnormal cholesterol levels."

Wow! For 20 years or more I avoided most foods with a high cholesterol content like eggs, butter, cheese, liverwurst—all foods I really loved and dearly missed. This left me eating a diet made up largely of carbohydrates, because they were the only foods not on the list of "don'ts."

For instance, being a creature of habit, especially for breakfast, every morning I had a bowl of Wheaties with non-fat milk with a sliced banana on top and a couple of pieces of toast and jelly—all carbohydrates—with decaf coffee. For the other meals, I ate chicken without the skin, some red meat, also pork, potatoes, pasta, egg beaters, bread, margarine, salads with low-fat dressings and low-fat cookies or low-fat ice cream for dessert.

I suffered through those 20 years. I like to enjoy what I eat, but I didn't enjoy the food doctors and food companies were pushing through the media to people like me with cholesterol problems.

"We're made out of protein, fats and cholesterol," Dr. Schwarzbein is quoted as saying in the *News-Press* article. "Cholesterol isn't evil. Any food with caloric content can turn into cholesterol. Our body says 'I need cholesterol.' If we don't eat it, the body says, 'I'll make it by turning carbohydrates into sugar, then into cholesterol.'"

She also warned in the article, "lest anyone misunderstand," that she is *not* saying high cholesterol in the blood does not lead to heart disease. "What I am saying," she emphasizes, "is that eating foods high in cholesterol does *not* increase blood cholesterol levels. I am saying that overeating carbohydrates can lead to abnormal cholesterol levels."

The solution, she believes, is very simple: "Eat a balanced diet of the four basic food groups: carbohydrates (breads, pasta, rice, etc.), protein (fish, poultry, meat, etc.), fat (butter, oil, cream cheese, etc.) and non-starchy vegetables (broccoli, cabbage, lettuce, etc.). It is important to eat something from each food group at every meal," she stresses.

Dr. Schwarzbein clearly had the credentials, as the head of the Endocrinology Institute of Santa Barbara, to know what she was talking about, so I decided to give her balanced diet a try.

I discussed my plan with my doctor. He was aware of Dr. Schwarzbein as a non-traditionalist in the medical field, and he lifted his eyebrows when I told him I was going to follow her diet. But he didn't advise me not to do it.

It took a lot of faith for me to follow Dr. Schwarzbein's balanced diet and believe it would help my cholesterol problem, as well as help me keep off the ten pounds I had lost when I was so very ill. I would now be eating some of the foods I loved but had been avoiding — food containing cholesterol and fat, such as eggs, butter, cheese, sausage and salads with real dressings. I hadn't eaten an egg, other than what Dolores used in cooking, for over twenty years, and I loved eggs. I loved liverwurst, which was high in cholesterol, and was delighted to look forward to eating a liverwurst sandwich once again.

I was sure that before my new balanced diet I had been overeating carbohydrates. Now, in order to cut down on carbohydrates and eat more protein, I would have to replace my Wheaties, banana, toast and jelly for breakfast. I checked a "food count" book to determine which foods are primarily made up of carbohydrate, protein or fat, and also to find out how many grams of each food group were in the particular food. I discovered that low-fat cottage cheese was high in protein but low in fat. I didn't particularly like cottage cheese, but mixed with cantaloupe or other fresh fruit, I didn't mind it. I then substituted natural peanut butter (no sugar added), which has a lot of fat in it—but *unsaturated* fat, the "good" kind. I spread this on my whole-wheat toast instead of jelly.

As I said before, I am a creature of habit. I ate this new breakfast about five times a week for the next year. I like to eat a substantial breakfast and have always thought that breakfast is the most important nutritional meal of the day. The other two days a week I splurged and ate eggs with buttered toast, sometimes adding ham or sausage.

For lunch, I'd have a salmon sandwich. I liked cold salmon right out of the can. Or I'd have a tuna salad or a ham sandwich on whole-grain bread. I was surprised to learn in the food count book that some ham is quite low in fat.

For dinner, I ate the usual balanced meal of vegetables, chicken, fish, pork or red meat and potatoes. I was in seventh heaven with this diet compared to what I had eaten the past 20 years.

At the start of this new diet, I went to the doctor for my yearly physical. My total cholesterol count was 250 (my doctor considered 240 borderline-high). He said I didn't have to worry how high my total cholesterol is as long as the HDL ("good cholesterol") was also high, because it's the ratio that counts. My HDL was 55, which, when divided into the total cholesterol, gave me a ratio of 4.5. The normal ratio my doctor wanted me to have was 3.5 or lower. I planned to stay on my new balanced diet for the next year until I had my next physical to see if the new diet would bring the ratio down.

Ten months later I had another physical. My total cholesterol dropped to 244 from 250, and my HDL good cholesterol was up to 60 from 55. My ratio was now down to 4.1. These results made a believer out of me. My doctor was very pleased, and so was I.

Four years after the start of my new balanced diet, I had my fifth and most recent physical exam. Results showed my cholesterol count had gone up to 269 from 250, an increase of 19 points. But my HDL also went up 19 points from 55 to 74, accounting for every one of the 19 point increase. My ratio was now down to 3.6. Again, my doctor was astonished and as pleased as I was. I was now practically in the normal range, which was 3.5 or lower.

My new balanced diet was a success. The doctor was also pleased that my weight had stayed the same at 170 over the four years. I had eaten the foods I loved, lots of food with fat, and kept off the ten pounds I'd lost when I was ill. I didn't measure my food or count calories, ate as much as I wanted, and never got hungry between meals. That's heaven!

High-Carb, Low-Fat Diets are Killing Us

These words screamed out from the headline of the *News-Press* interview with Dr. Schwarzbein when I came across it five years ago. At first, I thought this was an exaggeration to get the reader's attention. It certainly got mine. As I read on, I wanted to believe her. Now, after following Schwarzbein's recommendations for these past years, I credit her diet for the drastic decrease in danger of me having a heart attack or a stroke from too much cholesterol.

In the article, Dr. Schwarzbein also speaks about the impact of a high carbohydrate diet on weight gain and disease. "Not only are there more diseases today, but people are actually aging and dying because of high carbohydrate, low-fat diets," she reports.

Dr. Schwarzbein continues: "Low-fat diets are the enemy because they are usually low in both calories and protein (and high in carbohydrates), and lead to muscle loss and low metabolism. The whole irony is that people go on this diet because they are overweight or to prevent heart disease or to lower their cholesterol. Instead, they end up fatter and still get heart disease. In the past decade, we have become eight percent fatter.

"Heart disease statistics are even more disturbing," she states. "It's true that the death rate from heart disease has come down, but the incidence has increased. We're not preventing heart disease, only the death rate, and that's due to other factors like 911 responses, or procedures such as angioplasty or bypass operations."

The article describes how Schwarzbein began to question the value of the high-carbohydrate, low-fat diet while a medical student at the University of Southern California's School of Medicine and at Los Angeles County Hospital, which is affiliated with the school. Now she is board-certified as both an internist and endocrinologist, and she specializes in the treatment of the body's hormonal system.

"Hormones," she says, "are the chemical communicators of the body. They tell the heart and liver and other organs what to do."

While in training, Schwarzbein repeatedly saw patients with the same "cluster" of four symptoms — obesity, high blood pressure, high cholesterol and heart disease.

"They also had something else in common — scars down the middle of their chests from bypass surgery," she says. "Dr. Gerald Reaven of Stanford University names the cluster of symptoms *Syndrome X.*"

Schwarzbein wondered if there was a relationship between these symptoms, and if so, what it was. Did it have anything to do with insulin levels? Answers began to emerge in 1991 when she finished her residency and came to Sansum Medical Clinic in Santa Barbara to start a diabetes clinic.

"Patients were coming to me with the same four problems," she says, "but I wasn't seeing that the diabetes came first. They always came because of weight problems or cholesterol problems."

Schwarzbein was also alarmed by the increasing number of Type II diabetic patients, those who develop diabetes as adults. Type II diabetes occurs when the body is flooded with sugar.

"This overproduction of sugar can be caused by diet when patients overeat carbohydrates," she explains. "Usually insulin, a hormone, brings blood-sugar levels down. In Type II diabetes, the problem occurs when insulin can't get sugar, an energy source, into the muscle cells because the muscle cells can't accept any more sugar. Instead, the sugar moves on to fat cells, where it is either accepted or rejected. If rejected, it's then dumped into the blood stream, raising the overall sugar level in the body."

She began to zero in on insulin as a fat-storing hormone that causes the body to store fat, sugars and proteins as fat.

"Insulin is mainly secreted when carbohydrates are ingested," she states, "and protein stimulates some insulin release. Fats do not stimulate insulin release. Without insulin release, you cannot store fat as fat.

"Fat eaten with sugar," she explains, "is very fattening, but fat eaten with protein is not. For example, ice cream, which is a combination of sugar and fat, is very fattening. The reason is that sugar stimulates insulin release, and insulin will then take the sugar and fat and store it as fat. On the other hand, if you eat chicken with skin, which is a combination of protein and fat, the insulin levels stay lower and the body uses the protein and fat to build cells.

"In other words," she says, "insulin is like a chemical switch. Turn it up, and it stores energy as fat. Turn it down, and it signals the body that food is available and can be used to burn energy."

The solution, she believes, is very simple — eat a balanced diet of the four basic food groups (as mentioned before) — carbohydrates, protein, fat, and non-starch vegetables. Schwarzbein believes one serving of fat with meals is "desirable."

When she asks patients about their typical daily diet, they usually list a breakfast of non-fat cereal like Grape Nuts or Shredded Wheat with non-fat milk, a banana or orange juice and coffee with milk and sugar.

"The whole breakfast is sugar," she points out. "By 10 AM, they are starving, so they have a piece of fruit or a cappuccino or more coffee with sugar and milk," she says.

"A typical lunch will be a salad with non-fat dressing, a whole wheat roll with no butter and iced tea with artificial sweetener. To stave off fatigue in the late afternoon, they drink more coffee and eat snacks of rice cakes, low-fat pretzels or non-fat yogurt—all which have high levels of sugar to make them more palatable. Dinner is when the pasta comes out. Pasta and olive oil is the big thing now. Occasionally, they have fish or chicken, salad, again with non-fat dressing and wine or beer.

"All they've had all day is sugar. No wonder they complain about fatigue and weight gain. And foods that raise insulin levels are the ones that cause obesity, high blood pressure, high cholesterol and heart disease. Insulin levels should be normal, not too high nor too low."

Schwarzbein is particularly concerned about teen-agers who have grown up on the high-carbohydrate, low-fat diet, which has been popular for the past 15 years.

"I'm starting to see girls who are having problems with obesity, painful menstrual cycles, acne and excess facial hair," she says. "This is happening because carbohydrates increase insulin secretion. Insulin makes the adrenaline gland secrete androgens, such as testosterone, which is responsible for the acne, facial hair and prevention of ovulation.

"Too many doctors are telling these young women to eat less fat to lose weight, to take birth control pills for their painful periods, to take Accutane for their acne and to have electrolysis for their facial hair. I say all they have to do is change their diets. It's all about nutrition. Why take a drug when you can correct the situation with nutrition?"

Dr. Schwarzbein with Nancy Deville recently published *The Schwarzbein Principle* and two cookbooks with recipes for establishing a balanced diet, one of which is for vegetarians (see reference section). I highly recommend these books.

It May Be True After All—Pasta Makes You Fat

There's even more corroborating evidence that high-carbohydrate, low-fat diets make you fat. In the literature my daughter brought home from Dr. Schwarzbein's office, I read a *New York Times* article entitled "Bye-bye Pasta, It's Been Fun." It reported that "some diet experts who have been extolling the health benefits of low-fat, high-carbohydrate foods are now backtracking." Starchy foods, the experts now suspect, may be actually contributing to obesity.

Several of these experts are quoted in the article, corroborating the information given in Schwarzbein's *News-Press* interview.

"In the 60's, starch was the enemy, then sugar, then salt, then cholesterol, then fat," says Cathy Nonas, the director of the Theodore Van Itallie Center for Weight Control at St. Luke's Roosevelt Hospital Center in Manhattan.

The article continues: "And now starch is looking like the enemy again. Weight-loss experts and obesity researchers are studying the role played by insulin (a hormone produced by the body to process sugar and starches like those found in white bread, pasta and processed 'nonfat' snacks) in weight gain.

"The pendulum of weight-loss wisdom is constantly swinging, leaving behind some lasting scientific fact and some misbegotten notions. Few researchers question the health benefits of a low-fat diet, but many are beginning to wonder if a high-carbohydrate regime is appropriate for everyone, particularly overweight people and the 'insulin-resistant,' those who overproduce insulin after eating sugar or starches. Researchers estimate that at least 25 percent of the United States population may be insulin-resistant.

"The insulin-resistant respond to starches or sugar by overproducing glucose, which in turn causes an overproduction of insulin, a hormone responsible for a wide range of metabolic activities including determining how much of the glucose will be used immediately as energy and how much will be stored as fat, the regulation of triglycerides and perhaps even the stimulation of appetite."

Dr. Dean Ornish, the author of *Eat More, Weigh Less,* is quoted as saying. "The more insulin your body produces, the more likely it is that you will convert dietary calories into body fat."

Dr. James Hill, the associate director of the Center for Human Nutrition and an obesity expert at the University of Colorado in Denver, commented: "We may have gone too far with the low-fat emphasis. In the last decade, Americans cut their fat intake from 36 percent of their average daily calories to 34 percent. Nevertheless, they also gained about eight pounds a person.

"People can get fat on a high-fat diet," Dr. Hill adds, "but people can get fat on a diet high in carbohydrates, too."

Dr. Stephen Gullo, a Ph.D. in psychology and director of the Institute for Health and Weight Sciences in Manhattan, who has treated 10,000 overweight patients, reported in the article that over the last five years the question he has been asked most frequently is "How did I gain weight on a low-fat diet?"

To answer this question, Dr. Gullo, along with other clinicians and obesity researchers, considered the fact that rather than replacing dietary fat with complex carbohydrates like vegetables and fruits, many were reaching for simple carbohydrates like starch and sugar.

This realization led some researchers to revisit the scientific literature about the functions of insulin and to suspect that many dieters may be insulin-resistant. In addition, new research detailing performance has provided more insight into how the hormone is used.

Dr. Richard Heller, a professor of pathology at Mount Sinai School of Medicine and author, with his wife, Dr. Rachel Heller, of *The Carbohydrate Addict's Diet,* made this point: "The majority of overweight people are insulin-resistant. Carbohydrates are the worst thing they can eat because it causes them to overproduce insulin, which stimulates appetite, encourages the production of body fat and, over the long term, has serious health implications."

Dr. Ornish added: "Many assume that *non-fat* means *non-fattening.*" Dr. Ornish's low-fat program advocates eating larger quantities of complex carbohydrates like vegetables but fewer simple carbohydrates like honey, sugar and white flour, or drinking alcohol.

"The week that Entenmann's rolled out its fat-free desserts, a number of our patients gained weight," Dr. Ornish reports. "They thought that as long as they were eating something fat-free, they could eat as much as they wanted."

"Low-fat doesn't necessarily mean low-calorie," reports Linda Garill, general manager of corporate affairs for Weight Watchers International in Jericho, New York. "But if they count fat grams along with fiber, particularly the fiber in fruits and vegetables, they get a leaner, healthier way of eating."

By now, you may be, as I was, convinced that eating a high carbohydrate, low-fat diet is not the solution for losing weight and staying healthy, but that eating a balanced diet is.

How I Strengthened My Immune System

A year after I began the Schwarzbein balanced diet to solve my cholesterol problem and keep my weight down, I purchased a book by Dr. Barry Sears, a medical researcher, called *The Zone.* Dr. Sears' book has been a best seller, with more than a million copies in circulation (see reference section). I highly recommend it.

What is "the Zone?"

"Simply put," Dr. Sears says, "it's the metabolic state in which the body works at peak efficiency."

And what do you think Dr. Sears' recommendations are to "get into the Zone?" Eat a balanced diet of carbohydrates, proteins and fats at every meal, and also at the two daily snacks he suggests, one in the late afternoon and one in the evening.

Dr. Sears' advice, when added to my successful experience with Schwarzbein's balanced diet, gave me the confidence to continue my diet of protein and fat along with a reduced portion of carbohydrates at every meal.

Dr. Sears states in his book that a low-fat diet usually means a low-protein diet, because many fats contain both fat and protein—for instance, eggs, cheese, cottage cheese, chicken (with skin), pork and beef. He says adding more protein to our diet increases our stamina and energy, and it builds our immune system which helps to ward off illness.

Reading this over today, I realize this is what

happened to me as a result of eating cottage cheese almost every morning as well as adding eggs, butter, cheese and more meat to my diet. I stopped getting ill. All this extra protein must have built up my immune system. Honestly, I haven't been sick with a cold or the flu or any other illness since the devastating illness I had almost five years ago.

As I mentioned earlier, prior to going on a balanced diet, I would get a cold or the flu several times a year. What a pleasure it's been to not have to put up with illness over these last five years. A few minor symptoms during the flu season, which Dr. Sears suggested might happen, is all I have had. Nothing serious. They were gone in a day or two. I'm assuming my future years will be just as free of illness as the last five have been, as long as I keep eating a balanced diet. And why wouldn't I continue? I'm back to eating the foods I enjoy that I was afraid to eat for the previous twenty years. I now find they are good for me.

Wouldn't it be wonderful if we could convince people to add more protein to their daily diets, and thereby dramatically cut the flu epidemics that plague us every spring?

My confidence with this new diet grew even more when I read in Dr. Sears' book about how the Stanford University swim team was able to dramatically increase their energy and stamina and produce some amazing results.

"Nineteen- ninety- two was an important year for both the Stanford swim team and for the individual athletes involved," Dr. Sears writes. "For the past two years, the University of Texas swimmers (both men and women), had consistently beaten the Stanford team badly in the NCAA swimming championships. At the time, the University of

Texas was considered the top swimming program in the country. As individuals, the Stanford athletes were also training in that same year to make the U. S. team that would compete at the 1992 Olympics in Barcelona."

Most of the Stanford swimmers were happy with the high carbohydrate diets many athletes followed at the time and did not follow Dr. Sears' Zone program of a balanced diet. But six of the Stanford swimmers who did follow the Zone-favorable diet faithfully qualified for the U. S. Olympic team. The same year, their team also wrested the NCAA title from the University of Texas, and at the Olympic Games in Barcelona that summer, Stanford swimmers won eight gold medals. In the course of these accomplishments, the Stanford swimmers set two new world records.

In his book, Dr. Sears says learning how to control hormonal responses to food is our passport to entering and staying in "the Zone."

"Food is far more important than just something you eat for pleasure or to appease your hunger," he says. "Rather, it is a potent drug that you'll take at least three times a day for the rest of your life. Once food is broken down into basic components and sent into the blood stream, it has a more powerful impact on your body — and your health — than any drug your doctor could ever prescribe. Every time you eat, you are taking very strong medicine, which can have a good, bad, or indifferent effect on your body for the next four to six hours.

"What is a Zone-favorable diet?" Dr. Sears asks. "It's a diet in which the balance of micronutrients, like protein, carbohydrates and fat is tightly controlled. Every meal and every snack you eat should have the desired balances of micronutrients — protein, carbohydrates and fat — that produces an appropriate and favorable hormone response.

"Weight loss has little to do with will power," he continues. "You need information, not will power. If you change what you eat, you don't have to be overly concerned about how much you eat. Adhering to a diet of Zone-favorable meals, you can eat enough to feel satisfied and still wind up losing fat — without obsessively counting calories or fat grams.

"You fatten cattle by feeding them lots and lots of low-fat grains," Dr. Sears adds. "How do you fatten humans? Same way — you feed them lots and lots of low-fat grain. So if you've been eating more pasta and bread (both made from grain) than ever before, and you're gaining weight, think about those grain-fed cattle the next time you sit down to a big plate of pasta.

"Carbohydrate hell is the source of your carbohydrate cravings — including the infamous sweet tooth — and the constant cycle of recurring hunger that goes with them. These cravings are hormonally driven by that high-carbohydrate meal or, more accurately, by a ratio of food that was too high in carbohydrates and too low in protein.

"If you find yourself hungry and craving sugar or sweets two or three hours after a meal, you probably consumed too many carbohydrates that last meal," Dr. Sears warns. "Whenever you have a problem with hunger or carbohydrate cravings, look to your last meal for a clue to the reason why."

Endocrinologists find that the body has a tolerance for a certain quantity of protein and fat — only what the body needs. But they find that eating an excess of carbohydrates is like eating Cracker Jacks. "The more you eat, the more you want."

I conclude Dr. Sears' comments with the following startling statement: "The recommendations of the U. S. government in the food pyramid are dead wrong. The food pyramid, which has high-density carbohydrates as its base, will for many people be a prescription for elevated insulin, thus moving them further and further away from the Zone. If the base of the food pyramid were simply thrown away, you'd be left with a Zone-favorable diet."

Additional Thoughts About a Balanced Diet

As the saying goes, if you want to watch the game, you need a program. The program that you will need for setting up your balanced diet is a good "food count" book. The best-selling one, and the one I recommend is Corinne Netzer's *The Complete Book of Food Counts* (see reference section). In it, you can find the number of grams of carbohydrates, protein and fat in any of the foods you might like to add to your diet. I found cottage cheese as a good source of added protein. You may find other foods you prefer.

I don't recommend that you weigh or measure your food, nor weigh yourself to see how you are doing on your balanced diet. We got rid of our bathroom scale. You can tell how you are doing on your balanced diet by how your clothes fit. I check my belt. There's a certain hole in the belt that tells me I'm keeping off the ten pounds I lost five years ago. When I started to eat more proteins and fats in my diet, I found I didn't get hungry between meals. So if my belt gets a little tight, I cut down on the quantity of food I'm eating and I find I still don't get hungry.

On the cruise Dolores and I went on last year, I gained what I figured was about five pounds—one notch on my belt. In several weeks of eating a little less at each meal, I was back to my usual belt notch.

And remember, it is important to have some carbohydrate, protein and fat each time we eat, even for the two snacks a day allowed. The idea is not to eat a lot of food at one time, and you don't have to, if you can eat five times a day.

What about desserts? My favorites were hot fudge sundaes, or apple or cherry pie—all loaded with sugar, which is the worst of the carbohydrates. But believe it or not, and I hope you come to believe it, if you get enough protein and fat in your diet, you will slowly lose your craving for sweets. I did. I don't even have low-fat cookies in the house anymore, and I don't miss them.

Diatery experts believe that trans-fatty acids, the oil in which french fries, donuts, corn and potato chips are fried, may be even worse for your heart than saturated fat. But we have no way of knowing how much of it is in these foods. FDA commissioner Jane Henney is proposing that the amount of trans-fat be added to the amount of saturated fat on product labels. The move comes in the wake of research offering damning evidence against trans-fat, possibly the worst artery clogger of all. Studies indicate eating trans-fat increases LDL cholesterol, also known as "bad cholesterol" which increases the risk of heart disease. At the same time, it decreases the amount of HDL – the "good cholesterol" that is good for your heart. I have cut all of these foods out of my diet. The best way to get junk food out of your life is to not bring it home from the store. Now, in place of these high carbohydrate trans-fatty foods, I may eat lightly salted peanuts or almonds, or an apple with cheese for a snack. We usually have a late dinner, so sometimes I have non-fat crackers spread with cheese before dinner, or an apple with cheese, or celery spread with peanut butter or cheese. This way, even the snacks I eat are a combination of carbohydrates, protein and fat.

I still eat a high-carbohydrate dessert occasionally, usually if I'm out to dinner at a restaurant or at a friend's home. I try not to impose my diet on other people. If I go off the diet for a meal or a day, I simply go back on it again, without any guilt feelings. I don't believe in being a slave to a diet.

CAUTION! In adjusting food intake to lose weight, please be careful not to eliminate carbohydrates entirely from your diet. You may have heard of the high protein fad diets that do just that. Eating all protein and fat and little or no carbohydrates can cause *ketosis*, a serious abnormal state which can starve your brain and body of the daily carbohydrates they require. Always be sure you eat a minimum of 15 grams of carbohydrates (equivalent to one slice of whole-wheat bread or five saltine crackers) at each of the five meals and snack times allowed per day, adding up to no less than 75 grams per day.

When I told my brother about the balanced diet, he said he was afraid to cut out some of the cereals and pastas from his diet, because he believes he needs them to stay regular. So I sent him several tablets of Swiss Kriss Tabs to try. This is a gentle herbal laxative you can buy in a health food store which contains finely powdered sun-dried strawberry and peach leaves plus other natural herbs. I take one tab, rather than the two recommended on the bottle, and that works for me. Of course, I take it only on a day I'm constipated, before I go to bed that night. The next day I'm okay again—and now, so is my brother. I also find I have eliminated my hemorrhoids by taking these tabs, because now that I no longer have bowel problems, my hemorrhoids have healed.

While we're talking about little things that mean a lot in our lives, I thought about a problem of dryness in my nose that had bothered me since I was a kid. My nose would become uncomfortable and start to bleed. I told my doctor about it, and he recommended I buy a product that comes in a spray bottle called Ocean at any drug store. Now, especially when I visit our children in Santa Fe, New Mexico, where it is very dry, I bring my little bottle of Ocean along and use it whenever my nose feels dry.

I'm extremely satisfied, and so is my doctor, with the results of the balanced diet I've had over the four years between my first and last physical examinations. In addition to the positive cholesterol reports, I've kept off the ten pounds I lost through my last illness. I'm also very pleased my immune system is strengthened, and I haven't had to deal with getting sick in the past five years.

We had a family gathering recently with our eight children and their families, and Dolores and I celebrated our 55th wedding anniversary. They were all amazed at my energy and stamina. I am, too.

Chapter 5
Change Your Self-Image and Overcome Your Fears

In several instances in this book and in my previous book, *King of the Gumballs,* I have referred to my life-long struggle with self-consciousness and insecurity.

If there is one thing I could put my finger on that has kept me from attaining complete happiness in my life, it would be the insecurity I experience when relating to people I don't know. In spite of running a successful business for fifty years and working in various church organizations at the local and national levels, I still feel self-conscious when I have to interact in a group of strangers.

When I first began my peanut vending machine business at the age of 18, I was afraid to approach business owners about placing vending machines at their places of business, even though it would cost them nothing. I got around this obstacle by having others make the business contacts I feared doing myself. When the business grew beyond the peanut vending machines, I hired sales managers to do the selling of our various products, and so avoided having to talk directly to people myself.

I'm no longer in the vending machine business, but now, as a writer, I find myself facing the same obstacle of my social insecurity. In my new "business," I can't simply turn over the selling job of my books to other people. A distributor will handle the sales, but I'll be responsible for the promotion. Readers will want to talk to the author at bookstore signings, or listen to interviews with the author on radio and TV. The idea that I will have to talk to people brings up all my fears and self-doubts, and quite frankly, I'm scared to death even thinking about it.

In searching for a solution to my problem, I remembered a book I read 40 years ago that impressed me greatly. *Psycho-Cybernetics* by Dr. Maxwell Maltz dealt with teaching people to overcome their fears in communicating with others. Reading it over again, I wished I had done something years ago to alleviate my fears, instead of working around them as I did. But it's never too late to start, and I decided that if I can accomplish this now, not only will I be successful at selling my books, but I'll have less fear in all my communications, making my life more peaceful and happy. I looked on the bookshelves in our home and was pleased to find we still had the book, which is now out of print.

I was curious to find out if *Psycho-Cybernetics* would be as relevant today as it was when I first came across it, so I read it form cover to cover. I'm glad to say I was just as impressed today as I was then with the ideas presented by Dr. Maxwell Maltz, who wrote so many years ago.

The Power of the Self-Image

At the time he wrote *Psycho-Cybernetics*, Dr. Maltz was a famous plastic surgeon whose patients all suffered from some kind of disfigurement or deformity which they wanted corrected. He observed that most of his patients also had a poor self-image from having lived with their deformity, and that their poor self-image did not necessarily go away when their physical appearance changed.

In his search to understand more about this, Dr. Maltz discovered that people's images of themselves—good, bad or neutral—seemed to depend on whether they felt they had been successes or failures in their lives. "This concept," he says, "of one's own worth is so important, so much deeper and more meaningful than our image in a mirror. People carry this self-image of their own worth into their present activities, as well as their plans for the future."

Dr. Maltz continues: "To really *live*, to find life enjoyable, we must have a realistic, adequate self-image, one that we can accept. We must like and trust ourselves. We must feel that we can express ourselves without fear. We must feel no need to hide our true self. We must know ourselves well. And yet, our self-image must be realistic— who we really are. When our self-image is intact and adequate, we feel good about ourselves. We are full of confidence. We are ready to show the world what we are, and that we are proud of it. We breathe life, give deeply to it—and take happily from it.

"Make friends with yourself," Dr. Maltz urges us. "We must look beyond our physical features when we look into a mirror, to the inner face, emotions, beliefs, to the hidden stranger within us, which we cannot see in a mirror. *That* is our self-image. If it is an enemy, our self-image uses the failures of the past to undermine us, to make us a failure in the present. If it is a friend, our self-image draws from the confidence of past successes to give us courage to live and grow.

"Make friends with yourself!" he repeats. "Only then will you be happy and attain status as a human being! We are all unique. God did not mass-produce the human race. People do not roll off the assembly line like automobiles. God made people of different shapes and sizes and of different skin colors."

Dr. Maltz states that every person on earth, when compared to others, will find him or herself inferior in some way. We can't all golf as well as the professionals or act as well as the movie stars. Few can come near to having the compassion of Mother Theresa. The experience of feeling inferior usually happens because we have measured ourselves against another and then decided we are "not as good."

I recognized this way of thinking as the source of my own feelings of inferiority which I'd discovered some years ago when I attended a lecture in the "Mind/Supermind" series sponsored by Santa Barbara City College. The speaker had written a book about five different kinds of human intelligence he believed each of us has when we are born. He talked about how we choose our occupations on the basis of which of the five intelligences is more dominant in our make up. A person with *physical* intelligence, for example, might become an athlete, while another with *literate* intelligence might have a career as a writer, in business, or working with languages. *Spatial* intelligence would lead a person to a profession in the fields of geography, astronomy, and farming, while *mathematical* intelligence would dispose one to working with numbers and science. *Mechanical* intelligence covered the various building trades.

I felt good about myself when I left the lecture and went home that evening. What the speaker had talked about took the pressure off of me. I had been comparing myself to others and feeling inferior because I didn't measure up in every way. But now I could relax, because I saw that I didn't have to be good at everything, as long as I was good at one thing in my life. I felt I was good at business, and that was very satisfying.

It's not very likely that any one individual would excel in all areas of life. Even if someone did, there wouldn't be enough time to do it all. Besides, everyone benefits when some people specialize in one area over another. For instance, I am happy that some people have the skill to be plumbers. That's one job I really wouldn't like—climbing into dirty crawl spaces to fix people's toilets or water systems. I respect and admire any service person that comes to our home and repairs something I am unable to fix. Where would we be if we didn't have people to fix the toilet, the computer or the TV?

I think God was very resourceful when he handed out the different talents and skills, giving each one of us at least one special talent to develop and bring about fulfillment and happiness in our lives. Even those less fortunate than we, such as children with Down's syndrome, have a special talent. From what I have observed and heard from others, their particular talent is "exuding love," and that's an important one.

Knowing that I could do one thing well—business—was comforting to me, but it didn't completely solve the problem of my insecurity and self-consciousness. Reading *Psycho-Cybernetics*, I realized that I had some work to do in order to overcome my fears and gain the confidence to be comfortable and effective when talking to people.

I decided to develop a plan using the advice given by Dr. Maltz to change my self-image and deal with my fears. But before I take you through the steps of my plan, allow me to introduce you in more depth to the theory and practice of *Psycho-cybernetics*.

Self-Image and the Automatic Pilot

In his practice, Dr. Maltz found that most patients who had "freakish" features or conspicuously ugly faces experienced an almost immediate rise in self-esteem and self-confidence when their abnormality was corrected by surgery. However, many other patients did not come out of surgery feeling and acting better about themselves but continued to have the same poor self-image they had before surgery.

From this experience, Dr. Maltz came to an understanding that not all of a person's defects are visible, and that those which are not visible may be more difficult to change than the ones we can see, especially when they are deeply buried and infinitely painful. He observed that it was as if the personality, not just the body, had a "face"—a non-physical image held in the mind. He determined that this "face of the personality," or self-image, was the real key to changing the way a person felt and acted, and he wanted to find out exactly how this dynamic operated.

Dr. Maltz also believed that self-image, because it is

based in our sense of self-worth, sets the boundaries for our individual accomplishment. In short, it defines what we can and cannot do. Expand the self-image and we expand the "area of the possible." From this, he assumed that the development of an adequate, realistic self-image would imbue individuals with new capabilities, new talents, and literally, turn failure into success.

His search to understand more about how we can expand our potential took him beyond medicine to a new and emerging science, *cybernetics*. The study of cybernetics is concerned with the flow of information in both machines and human systems, and has been applied to the goal-oriented behavior of mechanical guidance systems, such as the automatic pilot in an airplane.

From his studies, Dr. Maltz observed that the human brain and nervous system operate in accordance with the known principles of cybernetics to accomplish the goals of the individual. On a functional level, he saw that the brain and nervous system constituted a marvelous and complex "goal-striving mechanism," similar to the built-in automatic guidance system that helps pilots fly planes. This mechanism works *for* us as a "success mechanism," or *against* us as a "failure mechanism," depending on what goals we set for it, and how we, the operators, use it. The science of cybernetics does not tell us that man *is* a machine, but rather that man *has* a machine available inside himself. Moreover, Dr. Maltz tells us how that machine functions and how we can use it most effectively.

Dr. Maltz proposed that every living thing, not only humans, has a built-in "goal-striving mechanism," an automatic pilot provided by the Creator to assure all creatures achieve their goals, whatever they may be. As I've heard it said, "God doesn't create junk!"

For animals, this built-in mechanism is limited to finding food and shelter, and avoiding or overcoming enemies and hazards—both activities aimed at insuring the survival of the species. A squirrel does not have to be taught how to gather nuts or how to store them for winter. Born in the spring, the squirrel has never stored nuts before, but it will do so before the winter, which it has never experienced before. A bird does not need to take lessons in nest-building, nor does it need to take courses in navigation. Yet birds do build nests and navigate thousands of miles, sometimes over the open sea where there are no visual cues for direction. The bird "knows" when cold weather is imminent and can find the exact location of a warmer climate, even though that location may be thousands of miles away.

In attempting to explain such things, we usually say animals have certain "instincts" which guide them. Analyze all such instincts and we find they assist the animal to successfully cope with its environment. In short, animals have a "success instinct" within them.

Scripture tells us that God created man and woman as a little less than the angels, and gave us dominance over the animals. While God endowed the animals with a goal-oriented mechanism for their success in self-preservation, he gave us the gifts of intelligence and creativity—gifts far beyond those given to the animals in value. How much more is possible for us, endowed not only with our human goal-oriented mechanism, but with the intelligence and creativity God has given us?

The Power of the Imagination

Dr. Maltz describes how we can use our creativity in conjunction with our goal-oriented mechanism. "Another item of equipment God has given us is our imagination. Imagination is as elusive as joy or sorrow. We can't put it in a bottle or get it out of one. It has no shape, and yet it gives us shape. Imagination is what puts the 'I' in 'Image.' It enters into our every act. It is imagination which gives us the goal for which we head; we act or fail to act. Our acts are accelerated or frozen because of our imagination.

"If we use our imagination positively, we can expand our horizons," he states. "In some schools of method acting, we find a wonderful example of imagination put to use. A method actor playing a king in a Shakespearean drama tries to think as if he were that king. He tries to put himself completely into this king's shoes. He stands on the stage and projects as if he were living the reality for the audience.

"But the use of imagination is not limited to the actor, or other creative artists," Dr. Maltz says. "We use it as they do—every day. Do you worry? If so, you are using your imagination—seeing yourself and imagining what can happen to you. Worry is a state of mind—before an event happens.

"Too many of us use our imaginations negatively— we worry. Not that worry doesn't sometimes have a positive function—it can prevent catastrophes, even save our lives. But many of us worry destructively. We stop our creative energies, keep ourselves from relaxing and continually imagine things that never happen.

"Let's take a common situation and see how you can use your imagination—positively or negatively—and what the results will be in each case. You work in an office. You've held down the same job for two years and you want a raise in pay. You're entitled to more money, you feel, since you've done good work. You have another child and you need the money. But you feel discouraged when you imagine what the boss's reaction will be.

"You picture the approaching interview in your mind. You'll knock timidly on his door—you always were afraid of the boss—and enter his private office. He'll be talking on the phone and signing letters at the same time and you'll sit down and wait for him to finish his phone call. You'll fidget in your chair and wonder if it's really such a good idea to ask for a raise—you could wait another six months, couldn't you? And, after all, he is such a busy man. You worry about what you should say first. Perhaps he'd be annoyed if you asked for a raise too directly. Maybe you should start talking about some neutral subject like the weather or....

"All right, do you think you would get the raise? I doubt it. Your imagination has betrayed you. You see yourself as a failure. And so you'll probably fail," he concluded.

As I read these words, I felt Dr. Maltz was talking directly to me. I have a very active imagination, and my problem is that I use much of it imagining bad things that never happen. For instance, when I imagine myself doing signings at a bookstore or talking to a group of people about my books, I see myself sitting very uncomfortably with my muscles tensed, terrified I'll forget the things I wanted to say.

I read on: "Now, let's put imagination to use again, but this time on your side. Once again, mentally picture the situation. You'll knock on the door of the boss. You won't smash it in, but you won't feel timid about it because you're asking for a raise that you know you deserve. You'll walk up to his desk, stride crisply and confidently, and sit down, waiting for him to finish his phone call. When he finishes, you'll ask him for your raise, knowing full well that you're worth every dollar you're asking for, and knowing that the boss realizes that, too. You are confident that you'll achieve what you're aiming at—your pay raise!

"Do you think you'll get it now? I do, because you are using your imagination to enhance your self-image. Put simply, you are betting on yourself! If we picture ourselves functioning in specific situations, it is nearly the same as the actual performance. Mental practice helps one to perform better in real life."

Dr. Maltz gives some examples: "A psychologist, using controlled experimental conditions, found that mental practice could help people throw darts more accurately. His subjects sat each day in front of the target imagining they were throwing darts at it. It improved their aim as much as actually throwing the darts. In another experiment, there were the effects of mental practice on improving skill in sinking basketball free throws. One group of students actually practiced throwing the ball every day for 20 days, and were scored on the first and last days. A second group was scored on the first and last days, and engaged in no sort of practice in between. A third group was scored on the first day, then spent 20 minutes a day, imagining that they were throwing the ball at the goal. When they missed they would imagine that they corrected their aim accordingly.

"The first group, which actually practiced 20 minutes

every day, improved their scoring by 24 percent. The second group, which had no sort of practice, showed no improvement. The third group, which practiced in their imagination, improved their scoring by 23 percent!"

I was fascinated to read how this same principle of using imagination to achieve a goal could also work in business. Dr. Maltz writes about a salesman who was doing so poorly selling his products that he considered changing occupations. He decided to go to a sales training seminar to see if he could find the solution to his problem. The instructor suggested he practice selling first in his imagination by thinking of every possible question or objection his customers could come up with, and having an answer in his mind for it. He practiced this daily for a period of time until he was so well versed in the selling of his products, he was able to relax with customers and no longer panicked when trying to come up with an answer. He could easily recall all the answers he needed to sell his product, and he went on to be a very effective salesman.

Dr. Maltz warns us that real change may need to go deeper. "The unhappy, failure-type personality cannot develop a new self-image by pure will power, or by arbitrarily deciding to do so. There must be some grounds, some justification, some reason for deciding that the old picture of self is in error, and that a new picture is appropriate. You cannot merely imagine a new self-image, unless you feel that it is based upon truth. Experience has shown that when people do change their self-image, they have the feeling that for one reason or another they 'see' or realize the truth about themselves.

"Science has now confirmed what philosophers,

mystics, and other intuitive people have long declared: Every human being has been literally 'engineered for success' by the Creator. Every human being has access to a power greater than themselves.

"This means *us*, "Dr. Maltz emphasizes. "If we are engineered for success and happiness, then the old picture of ourselves as unworthy of happiness, as a person who was 'meant' to fail, must be in error.

"We must learn to trust our creative mechanism to do its work and not 'jam it' by becoming too concerned or too anxious as to whether it will work or not, or by attempting to force it by too much conscious effort. We must 'let it' work, rather than 'make it' work. This trust is necessary because our creative mechanism operates below the level of consciousness, and we cannot 'know' what is going on beneath the surface. Moreover, its nature is to operate spontaneously according to present need. Therefore, you have no guarantee in advance. It comes into operation as you act and as you place a demand upon it by your actions. You must not wait to act until you have proof—you must act as if it is there, and it will come through. 'Do the thing and you will have the power,' said Emerson.

"As stated earlier, this new concept does not mean that *you* are a machine, but that your physical brain and body function together as a machine which *you* operate. This automatic creative mechanism within you can be operated in only one way. It must have a target to shoot at. You must first clearly see a thing in your mind before you can do it. When you do see a thing in your mind, your creative 'success mechanism' takes over and does the job much better than you could do it by conscious effort or 'will power.'

"Instead of trying hard by conscious effort to do the thing by iron-jawed will power, and all the while worrying and picturing to yourself all the things that are likely to go wrong, you simply relax the strain, stop trying to 'do it' by strain and effort, picture to yourself the target you really want to hit, and 'let' your creative success mechanism take over. Thus, mental-picturing the desired result, literally forces you to use 'positive thinking.' You are not relieved thereafter from effort and work, but your efforts are used to carry you forward to your goal, rather than in futile mental conflict which results when you 'want' and 'try' to do one thing, but picture to yourself something else.

"Picture yourself vividly as defeated, and that alone will make victory impossible. Picture yourself vividly as winning, and that alone will contribute immeasurably to success. Great living starts with a picture, held in your imagination, of what you would like to do or be.

"Your present self-image was built upon your own imagination pictures of yourself in the past which grew out of interpretations and evaluations that you placed upon experience," Dr. Maltz continues. "Now you are to use the same method to build an adequate self-image that you previously used to build an inadequate one.

"Set aside a period of 30 minutes each day when you can be alone and undisturbed," he advises. "Relax and make yourself as comfortable as possible. Close your eyes and exercise your imagination. Many people find they get better results if they imagine themselves before a large movie screen, imagining that they are seeing a motion picture of themselves. The important thing is to make these pictures as vivid and as detailed as possible. You want your mental pictures to approximate actual experience as much as possible. The way to do this is pay attention to small detail—sight, sounds, objects—in your imagined environment.

"One of my patients was using this exercise to overcome her fear of the dentist. She was unsuccessful until she began to notice small details in her imagined picture—the smell of the antiseptic in the office, the feel of the leather on the chair arms, the sight of the dentist's well-manicured nails as his hand approached her mouth, etc. Details of the imagined environment are all-important in this exercise, because for all practical purposes, you are creating a practice experience. And if the imagination is vivid enough and detailed enough, your imagination practice is equivalent to an actual experience, insofar as your nervous system is concerned.

"The next important thing to remember is that during this 30 minutes, see yourself acting and reacting appropriately, successfully, ideally. It doesn't matter how you acted yesterday. You need not try to have faith you will act in the ideal way tomorrow. Your nervous system will take care of that in time—if you continue to practice. See yourself acting, feeling, 'being' as you want to be. Do not say to yourself, 'I am going to act this way tomorrow.' Just say to yourself, 'I am going to imagine myself acting this way now—for 30 minutes—today.' Imagine how you would feel if you were already the sort of personality you want to be. If you have been shy and timid, see yourself moving among people with ease and poise—and feeling good because of it. If you have been fearful and anxious in certain situations—see yourself acting calmly and deliberately.

"This exercise builds new 'memories' of stored data

into your mid-brain and central nervous system, Dr. Maltz advises. "It builds a new image of self. After practicing it for a time, you will be surprised to find yourself 'acting differently', more or less automatically and spontaneously — 'without trying.' This is as it should be. You do not need to 'take thought' or 'try' or make an effort now in order to feel ineffective and act inadequately. Your present inadequate feeling and doing is automatic and spontaneous because of the memories, real and imagined, you have built into your automatic mechanism. You will find it will work just as automatically upon positive thoughts and experiences, as upon negative ones."

My Plan

As I mentioned earlier, I was so inspired by Dr. Matlz's words, I decided to try the method described in *Psycho-Cybernetics* to solve my life-long problems of insecurity and self-consciousness. With the help of my very active imagination, I know I can cultivate the positive thoughts I need to talk confidently about my book at book signing events and for interviews on radio and TV shows. So, here goes!

First, I find a quiet corner where I will be undisturbed. Then I begin to imagine myself in exactly the way I want to be. I picture myself in the new Barnes & Noble bookstore at the Fox River Mall in Appleton, Wisconsin, where I have arranged for a book signing shortly after publication in the year 2000. New century, new me!

I see myself confidently walking into the book store and asking for Mary, the event coordinator I spoke with on the phone. After checking in with her, I go to my car and get the boxes of books Mary suggested I bring. I also have extra books in my car, in case sales are higher than Mary anticipated.

I ask Mary to have chairs set up so people can sit while I address the group. If the group is small, I won't be disappointed, but will talk casually with them and others when they come in during the period for which I'm scheduled. If there are a dozen or more coming in, I talk to them confidently and get a discussion going about the book.

But before things begin, I see myself sitting at a table with a few stacks of my books placed on it and more in a box underneath. I'm at the book store early enough so that I'm not rushed. Enjoying the fine aroma of the Starbuck's coffee I bought at the store's cafe, I continue to visualize my successful day until people arrive, feeling confident that what I have written is informative and interesting to them.

I see myself as relaxed and mentally prepared to come up with the appropriate remarks when I communicate with people. I tell them how the book describes the many ways people can bring more health and happiness into their lives. I also relate the clever comment a friend of mine made on the phone when I told him the title, *Listen to Your Body and Add 10 – 15 Years to Your Life*. "I'll be happy to spend $9.95 for ten extra years," he said, laughing.

I'm prepared beforehand to talk about specific chapters I feel will be the most interesting to people, and am well-versed in my material. I don't consciously try to remember what I want to talk about. I see myself relaxed, having a good time and letting go of any preconceived ideas of what I might do or say, just letting the event unfold naturally.

I imagine talking to people as if they are all like my

good friend Tom, a person I am always comfortable with and can say anything to without being afraid of his response. I am completely at ease. If I find myself getting tense, I take a deep breath and relax my arms or whatever part of my body feels tense. I keep the conversation light and let my natural humor come out.

As I sit at the table, I continue to feel that everyone who buys a book will love it. I ask people if they'd like to purchase my book and am not offended if they decline because they just came to hear about it. If they do purchase a book, I make sure to ask them their first name and write it on the cover page. Then I sign my name and give them the book. I thank them for coming and thank them again if they purchased a book, and ask them to tell others about it.

And that's it!

On re-reading this step by step exercise I've just gone through, I must admit I feel a bit foolish. Talking to people at a bookstore about a book I have written should be a simple thing to do. But now, having done this exercise, when I think about doing a book signing, I no longer feel the apprehension I felt before. Instead, I feel confident that I can talk with people without feeling insecure and self-conscious. I figure if I've made this much progress simply writing about the situation, I should have much more confidence after I practice mentally in the months ahead. The first bookstore event should go well and future ones be routine.

I am still afraid at the prospect of doing radio and TV interviews if I want to introduce my book to people across the country. But I'm comforted that the bookstore event already seems easier as a result of the short time I spent imagining it. I'm sure the interview situation will also be easier after I "do it" in my imagination umpteen times. And once I've mastered book signings and media interviews, I can begin to work on feeling confident in other situations in my life. I know I've got a lot of mental practicing to do to conquer my insecure feelings, but if having more self-confidence adds to my happiness, which I know it will, the effort will be well worth it.

I hope my experience of imagining a positive response to a challenging situation is helpful, especially if you, like me, have fears that stop you from having everything you want out of life.

Chapter 6
Exercise At Home In Only 10—15 Minutes a Day

I thought of titling this chapter "Exercise for Dummies—like me, who don't exercise regularly." This is one area where I fall down in my own health program. I congratulate those of you who exercise regularly. Keep it up.

For those of us who know we should exercise regularly but don't, I have worked out an exercise program with the help of my daughter, who is a physical education instructor. She feels these are some of the best exercises in the California school system.

You can do these exercises in your home in 10 or 15 minutes a day without the need of any exercise equipment. It will not only exercise your upper and lower body, but it will give your back and heart a good workout, as well.

But first a word of caution: If you have had any recent physical problems or surgery, particularly of the heart, joints or muscles, or if you have been inactive or sedentary for some time, please consult your physician before you start doing these exercises.

Be kind to your body. Start this exercise program at the lower levels recommended and gradually increase the time you spend on each exercise. That is why you may need only 10 minutes to complete the exercises at first and up to 15 minutes to complete it later on.

This program consists of primarily stretching exercises. Why stretch? Because it relaxes your mind and tunes up your body. It releases muscle tension, increases your range of motion, helps to prevent injuries, such as muscle strain. It also makes strenuous activities easier and develops body awareness. As you stretch various parts of your body, you focus on them and get in touch with them. You get to know yourself better. Also, it promotes circulation, and most importantly, it feels good.

If you stretch correctly and regularly, you will find that every movement you make becomes easier. It will take time to loosen up tight muscles. Be patient. Time is quickly forgotten when your muscles feel good.

When you begin a stretch exercise, spend up to 30 seconds holding the stretch, as noted in the instructions below. Go to the point where you feel mild tension. Relax and breathe as you hold the stretch. The feeling of tension should subside as you hold the position. If it does not, ease off slightly and find a degree of tension that is comfortable. If you experience pain, you have gone too far—ease off.

At first, silently count the seconds recommended in the instructions for each exercise. By counting 1001, 1002, etc., you can determine the number of seconds elapsed. After a while, you will be stretching by the way it feels, without the distraction of counting.

Here are the seven exercises that make up the

program:

No. 1—WARM UP EXERCISES—1 minute

a) Stand up straight, shoulders relaxed, chest up.

b) Raise both your heels, placing weight on balls of feet, not on toes. Hold for three seconds (remember: 1001, 1002, 1003), then lower heels. Repeat up to 10 times.

c) Start with your feet flat on the floor and shoulder width apart. Raise your right heel, keeping toes on the floor. Keep your knees bent slightly. Then raise your left heel. Continue to alternate heels quickly, counting each time your left heel hits the floor. Do this for up to the count of 30.

d) With your feet flat on the floor, extend both your arms to the side and start rotating them clockwise, small circles first, then going to larger circles. Then rotate your arms counter-clockwise. Do this 30 times each way.

No. 2—STRETCHES FOR LOWER BACK AND HAMSTRINGS—1 minute

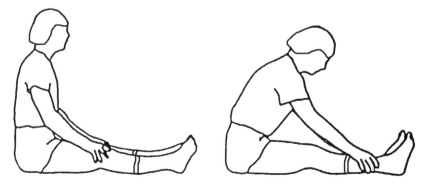

a) Sit up straight on a mat or carpeted floor or put

your back against the wall. Put your hands on your knees.

b) Move your hands forward on your legs, bending from the hips to a point where you feel mild tension (not pain). Hold position for up to 20 seconds. Try to keep your head and back in a straight line. Can be repeated two or more times.

No. 3—BACK MUSCLES AND HAMSTRINGS STRETCH—1 minute

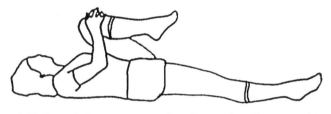

a) Relax, lying on your back on the floor and let your head rest on the floor.

b) Pull your left leg toward your chest, but don't strain. If you can't do it with your head down on the floor, that's okay. Keep the other leg as straight as possible, without straining. Hold your leg in this position for up to 30 seconds.

b) Do the same with the other leg. This will help to slowly loosen up the back muscles and hamstrings.

NO. 4—LOWER BACK STRETCH—1 minute

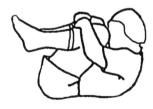

a) Lie on your back. Place your arms around your knees and gently pull your knees toward your head until they touch. Then gently roll around on your spine for 30 seconds, keeping your chin down toward your chest. This will further stretch the muscles along the spine. Exercise can be repeated.

NO. 5—QUADRICEP LEG STRETCH—1 minute

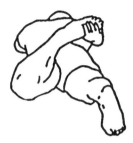

    a) Lie on your stomach. Reach behind you with your hand (or both hands if necessary) and grab your opposite foot between the ankle and toes. Gently pull your heel toward the middle of your buttocks. Hold for 8—12 seconds.

    b) Then do the same with your other foot. Exercise can be repeated.

NO. 6—ARM-MUSCLE STRENGTHENER—1 minute

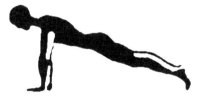

    a) Get into the position as above.

    b) Hold up your body with both arms. Pick up your left hand and touch your right shoulder, then put it back. Pick up your right hand and touch your left shoulder, then put it back. Repeat this up to 25 times, counting each time you touch a shoulder. Try it. It's easier than you think. Can be repeated.

NO. 7—HEART RATE EXERCISE —5 minutes.
CAUTION: If you are considerably overweight or have any heart problems, definitely talk to your doctor before doing this exercise.

a) This is a stationary run, meaning you run in place. Raise your right foot, then your left foot. Count a step each time your left foot touches the floor. Lift your feet approximately four inches off the floor.

b) Beginners try 300 steps or less, others up to 500 steps. This exercise can be replaced with a one or two mile walk if you have the time.

Good posture is an exercise you can practice all day long – every time you think about it. Imagine a string coming out of the middle of the top of your head and it is pulling your head and body up straight as far as it will go. Walk as tall as you can, eyes looking straight forward.

I tried these stretching exercises to determine whether they were okay for me. At the age of 76, having done very little exercise during my lifetime, I was not surprised how confined my movements were, especially compared to my daughter's. But doing the exercises also showed me how much I needed to be doing the program on a regular basis. I'm sure if I do these exercises faithfully, I will become more limber as I grow older. I don't want to end up a creaky old man, so I plan to continue them. How about you?

Chapter 7
Resolve the Negative Feelings Buried Deep Inside of You

Do you keep negative thoughts and feelings buried deep inside you, holding them down until they erupt and surface as anger, frustration, loneliness, fear, jealousy or depression?

Most of us have unresolved situations in our lives, such as the death of a loved one or fear of one's own death, broken or tarnished relationships with lingering hurts, an illness you or someone dear to you has suffered. These and other situations may have caused thoughts and emotions to be pushed below consciousness, because they are too painful to think about.

It's uncomfortable and frustrating to bring our negative feelings to mind, having learned from past experience that whenever we try to resolve them, we tend to wallow in our misery and go nowhere. The same negative feelings come up over and over again, never reaching any kind of resolution or relief. As a result, most people avoid getting too close to these difficult feelings, not wanting to experience the pain once again.

Years ago, I discovered a remarkable process that opened up an entirely new dimension in my life and helped me to deal with my own buried feelings. This process, called *Focusing*, taught me that we can tap into our body's wisdom to resolve problems and concerns not resolvable through the mind alone.

A Focusing Adventure

In 1975, Dolores and I packed up our furniture and belongings in Appleton, Wisconsin, hired a moving van, and with our two youngest children, moved to Florida. I was escaping, hopefully forever, the Wisconsin winters which I had detested since I was a youngster.

A few weeks after we arrived in Florida, we got a call from Father Myron, a priest and friend of ours in Wisconsin. He told us about a weekend workshop that was being offered in Racine on Focusing, a process that taught people how to resolve their deeply buried negative feelings on an ongoing basis. He said the process could be learned in a weekend by those attending a Focusing workshop, although it would take some time to integrate it in one's life as a habit.

It sounded too good to be true. Ten years before, I had spent thousands of dollars for two years of psychotherapy sessions with a psychiatrist, not because I was mentally ill, but because I lacked self-esteem. I was insecure and uncomfortable dealing with people one-on-one in the business world, and I knew this would have to change if I were to succeed in the challenges of running my own business. I was helped greatly by the therapy, and, at the time, I felt it was the best money I'd ever spent. Now, hearing about Focusing, it was hard to believe that people could administer this type of therapy to themselves without the aid of a therapist. I had to see it for myself, so Dolores and I flew back to Wisconsin for the workshop, which began on a Friday.

Father Myron had arranged for an informal meeting with the two workshop facilitators before the workshop began. Ed McMahon and Peter Campbell, we learned, were Jesuit priests, both with doctorates in psychology, who were presenting the workshop. They impressed me as congenial, down-to-earth guys. Both had taught courses on the psychology of religion in the Department of Religious Studies at the University of Ottawa in Canada.

Ed and Peter filled us in on the background of how they came to lead Focusing workshops. While teaching at the university, they had become interested in the work of Dr. Eugene Gendlin, a professor in the department of psychology at the University of Chicago. Dr. Gendlin had been one of the psychologist Carl Rogers' early graduate students and was fascinated with his mentor's theories.

In his work at the University of Chicago, Gendlin made the observation that some people succeeded in therapy while others did not. He was determined to find out why this was so, and if those that succeeded had something in common that helped them to succeed.

As part of his research, Gendlin had his graduate students listen to short segments of taped interviews with patients who were in therapy. His students were able to predict with remarkable accuracy which patients would be successful. Those who were able to experience their problems as a sensation somewhere in their bodies were clearly the ones to benefit by the therapy. Gendlin called this experience of the successful patients a "felt-sense" — an awareness of how a person's body carries an issue, a kind of bodily knowing. From this information, Gendlin developed the self-help therapy he called Focusing.

Ed and Peter mentioned that by the time our Focusing workshop was over, Dolores and I hopefully should experience this felt-sense in our bodies, as well as what Gendlin called a "felt-shift" — a perceptible change in how the body carries an issue.

We continued listening as they explained how, after working with Gendlin's Focusing Institute for several years, they determined there was another dimension to Focusing, a surprise or gifting experience they believed to be God's grace. Gendlin agreed there was something missing in his process and was pleased to have Peter and Ed explore their theory of the grace dimension.

I was amazed to hear how these two new Focusing advocates had added their Christian tradition to Gendlin's Jewish tradition. They believed that the felt-shift which can sometimes happen in Focusing is actually the intervention of God's grace. They called their new approach *BioSpiritual Focusing*, a name that acknowledges the body's role in spiritual growth.

How Focusing Works

On the first day of the workshop, the 15 participants gathered in a school classroom to meet with Ed and Peter. Our leaders took their places at the front of the room and announced they would be working individually with each of us as the workshop progressed. First, however, they wanted to introduce us to Focusing and tell us what we could expect to get out of the experience. Peter, a thin, youngish, blond-haired guy, who seemed to smile often, spoke first.

"Do you ever get the feeling something is bothering you, but you can't put your finger on what it is?" he asked. Most of us could relate, and we nodded our heads in agreement.

He continued: "Have you ever met people who, 20, 30, even 50 years after they were wronged by some person or circumstance, still feel exactly the same way about the person or situation? When they tell their stories, they relive the entire episode again, and their hurt never changes. The old battle wounds remain unhealed.

"As children, many of us were never taught how to be present with our pain and negative feelings in a way that would allow them to unfold and feel better in our bodies. Instead of learning to 'be in our hurt,' we grew to think of painful feelings as something to be avoided, because they made our bodies feel bad. Some of us learned to distance ourselves from our feelings, to become good at distracting ourselves from the pain, and so created our own little protected worlds, sealed off from others.

"But there really is no way we can shield ourselves from events in our lives that may hurt us. Feelings of anger, jealousy, fear and guilt sweep over us as a natural reaction to many life situations. They simply happen."

The room was still as we listened and absorbed Peter's words.

"The problem is that now, as adults, most of us never allow our private hurts to unfold and be experienced fully. We develop a habit of denying that our hurt feelings even exist, burying them deep inside ourselves, which is what probably causes the distress we feel in our bodies. Eventually, we stop wanting to feel anything, for fear that what might come up will be all the old hurts that were never allowed to unfold in the first place. The price we pay for this is that we gradually shut down our ability to listen to our bodies.

"Deep down, though, our bodies know that those unprocessed experiences are still there. Each of us instinctively realizes this, and we are usually reluctant to get in touch with them. As a result, the idea of feeling anything at all becomes extremely risky for some people."

As I listened, I thought about my relationship with my father, which I usually kept buried inside myself, and I felt an uneasiness in my stomach. Peter continued.

"It's no wonder, then, that we go along experiencing life almost exclusively in our heads. We reject our bodily knowing which eventually takes its toll, and we suffer from physical and emotional breakdowns. As someone once said, mental illness is brought on not because we've gone 'out of our minds,' but because we've been 'in our minds' too much.

"Mother Theresa made an interesting observation that seems relevant. She said that society knows, in general, how to care for the hungry, the naked and the sick. But she was concerned about a far more radical poverty, especially in the West, that is subtle and more difficult to transform. Food, clothing and all the bandages in the world can never touch the frustration, anxiety, loneliness, anger, and depression that permeate our culture. This, she pointed out, requires a different kind of healing.

"What makes Focusing work is that it creates an inner

climate around our painful and frightening issues which is different from the climate we normally experience with our problems and difficulties. Usually, we feel bad—ashamed, guilty, annoyed or impatient—about things we don't like in ourselves. We hold our problems at arm's length and try to control what we cannot accept. Focusing invites us to relate differently to that which we perceive as unlovable in ourselves."

Peter then told us about an incident that occurred in a Focusing workshop he and Ed facilitated with Dr. Gendlin. "One of the participants made the point that she found it relatively easy to experience positive feelings of joy, excitement, love, tenderness, and curiosity. But when it came to anger, depression, guilt, loneliness, frustration, or a desire for revenge, she found it much more difficult, often impossible, to experience these emotions.

"Dr. Gendlin's response was to challenge her to adopt a new perspective. He said: 'You must learn to be with your negative feeling as you would be with a hurting child. Sit down with your hostility, fear, or grief, and deliberately put your arm around those things in yourself which for years you have held at arm's length. This is quite a challenge, but it can be done!' "

A Caring-Feeling-Presence

Ed, a robust gentleman with salt and pepper hair, and a goatee, spoke to the group next.

"I want to emphasize how important it is to be sympathetic to your negative feelings," he began. "I call this ability a 'caring-feeling-presence.' It's a kind of feeling that says to those lonely or confused places inside us, 'You are not alone. I'm here, and I care.'

"Those frightened places inside of us need to have this caring-feeling-presence communicated to them directly through our bodies, because too often we have made our fearful feelings into the enemy. In caring, we start to build a kinship with them. Trust begins to develop. Then they hang around more easily and we carry them in a different way. When the fearful feelings are no longer the enemy, we can begin to own them in our body. Sooner or later they will start to tell us their story, just like a friend who felt accepted might do. With that comes the processing and a change in feeling inside us. This is the object of the Focusing process."

Ed continued: "We all have experienced what this caring-feeling-presence is. When someone in the hospital is too medicated or weak to talk, we instinctively reach out with a hug or with our hand to say, 'I care and I'm here with you.' We know our body has to communicate the message if we want it to be heard. Similarly, when a toddler is frightened by the sudden lunge of a dog, we don't stop to explain about safety, but instead communicate our message by taking the child up in our arms and holding it close to us. We hold the scared infant differently, say, than we hold a bag of groceries. We know the tone of our voice, our open arms and warm chest have to do the talking for us, because the child needs to feel care and safety on a physical level.

"So, too, do those painful places inside us that we have rejected, neglected or disowned as the enemy. They need to feel our acceptance, openness, and availability—the caring-felt-presence—before there is a change in how they feel in our body.

"Affection is the body's way of surrendering, of letting

go, of being vulnerable and open," Ed continued. "Affection disposes our body, as well as our mind, to be changed. Through affection, there is an opening up to be penetrated by the object of our affection. For example, we allow another to bring tears to our eyes, caring to our touch, warmth to our embrace, gentleness to our voice, patience to our presence. We do not put up barriers to being touched or moved by the other. There is a letting go that happens when we respond with our body and our feelings, that doesn't happen when we respond only with our minds. A caring-feeling-presence, which always embodies some degree of affection, is the only way we can change our body's attitude toward these negative feelings inside us."

Ed concluded his talk with a short story:

"A grandmother came to visit her sick grandson. The little boy had just received a puppy for his birthday and wanted it on the bed with him during his recuperation. His mother wouldn't allow it, because the puppy had not yet been housebroken, and she was afraid it would do 'puppy things' on the bed. But the grandmother insisted the puppy stay with the boy, because, as she told the mother: 'He loves that puppy and will get well sooner if he can hold it near him.' She instinctively knew that the affection stirred up by the puppy in her grandson's body would speed up the healing process. By holding the puppy with affection, he would more likely hold his own pained body with affection, and his recovery would be enhanced."

His point having been well taken, Ed announced a lunch break. When we returned, we would be divided into two groups so he and Peter could lead us individually through the five-step Focusing process. He suggested that during our break, we take some time to try to feel the affection and caring-feeling-presence he talked about. It would be the most important ingredient in learning to do Focusing successfully.

The Five Steps of Focusing

Returning from the break, I was assigned to Peter's group and joined him in a quiet corner of the room. He and I sat on chairs facing each other. I was a little nervous wondering what was in store for me.

Peter started by saying that we would proceed through a series of questions he would ask. I was to answer, but not out loud. Instead, I would be answering his questions inside myself in silence. The Focusing leader, he explained, didn't need to know what the subject of the Focusing was, nor did he need to get involved in a discussion with the person doing the Focusing during any part of the process, unless there were questions about the procedure. I found this very comforting and was able to relax.

He told me there were five steps in the Focusing process, and I should indicate when I was ready to proceed to the next step by moving my right hand a little.

"The first step," he began, "is to take a few minutes to allow yourself to grow quiet inside and allow your attention to settle into the center of your body. Ask yourself, 'How am I feeling right now? Is there anything bothering me? Is there anything keeping me from feeling really good at this moment?' Then sit there with these questions for a while and sense how your body responds. Signal me when you want to proceed further."

Various problems came to mind. I thought about my

relationship with my father when I was growing up. I felt a tightening in my stomach. There were also some unresolved problems between Dolores and me. I had a problem with one of my employees. I thought about these concerns for a few minutes, then signaled I was ready for the next step.

"The second step," he continued," is to feel which of your issues is the one that is bothering you the most. To do this, imagine you are in a room on the second story of a building, looking out the window at the street below. Imagine that each of the issues or thoughts that comes up is a different vehicle going by in the traffic below. Wait for a big fire truck issue to come racing by with the horns sounding and lights flashing. That's the signal that you have found what's bothering you the most right now."

I understood immediately what Peter was saying. The fire engine appeared the minute I thought about my relationship with my father. It not only appeared in my imagination, but I felt it in my stomach as well. I moved my hand, letting Peter know I was ready to proceed further.

"The third step is to ask yourself this question: 'Is it okay to be with all that surrounds this issue inside me?'" He explained that sometimes very painful issues can come up, and if any were too painful to handle at this time, I should put them "on the shelf," so to speak, to revisit at a later date. He cautioned never to force the body to handle something it was not yet ready to handle.

I was glad he said that, because touching this issue of my relationship with my father frightened me. I figured I would need more experience with Focusing before I tackled a problem as deep as that one. I tried Focusing instead on my relationship with Dolores. After several minutes, nothing came up for me about that relationship, but I was aware of a feeling of fear about the Focusing process itself. That was a surprise to me, and, since this was a teaching session, I opened my eyes and told Peter what was going on.

"Then focus on your fear of Focusing," Peter suggested. "And ask yourself again: 'Is it okay to be with all that surrounds the feeling about this inside me?'

I let my fear of Focusing settle in, and after a few minutes I was aware of a lot of unresolved issues between Dolores and me. I was afraid to go into any of those issues, which was undoubtedly why I was experiencing the fear of Focusing. So I put the issues with Dolores "on the shelf," alongside the issues with my father, to touch on again at a later date.

Then I tested how it would feel to Focus on the problem I had with my employee. I let that sink in to see how it felt, and found it safe to focus on. I signaled Peter to let him know I was ready to go to the next step.

Peter continued. "Step four is a special way of getting beyond the tendency to hold what hurts you at arm's length. In this step, you let go into how your body is carrying the issue. If the main thing you're aware of about a painful feeling is wishing it would go away, then you'll always be one step removed from the actual feeling that needs to change. Transformation becomes possible to the extent that you directly touch the way you carry an issue and not just your resistance to it. This encourages an attitude of open listening to what is really inside you—the hurt, confusion, bitterness, longing, or whatever.

"Don't try to figure out the solution to the issue or problem that's bothering you," Peter added. "You've probably already tried that without success. In Focusing, simply be with what is real inside you in a caring way, not trying to fix or change anything. Take the time to let this place inside you know that you care enough just to be with it. You don't change it. It changes itself! When this happens, you will know how grace feels in your body.

"You may find it useful to follow the suggestion I told you Dr. Gendlin offered the woman who found it difficult to experience her negative emotions," Peter stated, "Imagine you are holding the painful issue just as you might hold a hurting child. In your imagination, put your arms around whatever part of your body you may be feeling the pain in, treating it with sympathy and kindness—the caring-feeling-presence Ed talked about earlier. Or use Ed's imagery of the affection you may have felt for a child, or the comfort of your favorite blanket or stuffed toy, or whatever feeling would be kind to the hurt feeling inside you. Then be with that hurt feeling for as long as you feel the need to do so. Let me know when you have touched this painful place inside you."

I tried the best I could to get out of my head and into my body, to surround the painful feeling inside me with all the love and caring I could muster. The sympathy, love and kindness I was giving to my body was certainly feeling good. When I had done this for several minutes, I moved my hand to show Peter I was ready to proceed.

The fifth and final step of the process was to allow the issue being Focused on to express itself in the body. Peter explained how this can happen.

"Given time and faithfully remaining in what we are feeling without trying to control the feeling or to force it in any way, we eventually are able to experience the inner meaning as it expresses itself to us. Sometimes a word or picture will suddenly appear to tell you what it is all about. It will often be a spontaneous image. Occasionally, there will be tears or irrepressible giggling to accompany the image. Some tangible symbol should eventually appear, often bringing with it a tinge of surprise.

"You immediately know the accuracy of a symbol by the distinct sense of inner release you feel in your body," Peter continued. "This is the resolution, and it always feels good. It's the 'felt-shift' Dr. Gendlin identified when he looked at why some patients are successful in therapy. It's a shift in the way your body is carrying the issue you are Focusing on."

I followed Peter's directions and stayed with that feeling in my body, keeping it warm and cozy while waiting for something to happen. It seemed like five minutes, but was probably less. And then, all of a sudden, the word "control" came to me, and I felt this was the word or symbol Peter was talking about. I realized that the problem with my employee was one of control.

With this new insight, I experienced an inner release, which I believed was the "felt-shift" in the way my body was holding the issue. It felt good, this letting go of the tightness I'd been feeling whenever I thought about my relationship with this employee. The issue with him hadn't changed, as Peter explained it wouldn't, but I no longer had that sick feeling in my stomach when I thought about it. I now knew what bothered me about my relationship with him. I felt controlled, and I didn't like it. I moved my hand to let Peter know I was ready to continue.

Peter told me I could open my eyes, as the Focusing process was now finished. He asked me whether I had experienced the felt-shift in my issue, and I told him I thought I had, and that it felt good. He asked me whether I had a better feeling about the issue than I'd had before the Focusing, and I told him yes, the discomfort I'd felt in my body due to the problem was gone.

Insights from Focusing

That night, I thought about the breakthrough I'd had in the workshop. I now understood the problem I had with my employee was about my feeling he was controlling me. With this new insight, I would be able to figure out what to do about it.

I also thought about my relationship with Dolores. I realized that "control" was also my issue with her. I wasn't sure who was controlling whom, but as I thought about it, I realized each of us was trying to control the other, and perhaps I more than she.

The issue of control also seemed relevant to the problems I had with my father. He tried to control me when I was growing up, and my body had rebelled against his efforts. I thought also about other control problems I had faced in my life, my unhappiness in grade school, where the nuns controlled me, and in the Army, where I had been expected to give blind obedience to the authority of my superiors. I didn't like being controlled, and having my own business, I'd grown accustomed to being the one in control.

Now, I had my future cut out for me. I was at least aware of the problem that was causing the negative feelings inside of me all these years, and I could do something about it. It would take me months and possibly years to Focus on these control issues and chip away at them piece by piece, until I could resolve them in my body, as well as in my mind.

I reflected on what Peter had told the group that day, that even though we may not get a complete healing the first time we Focus on an issue, each succeeding time, it would be less scary, and eventually resolve itself completely and leave us at peace.

The group met again on Saturday morning and we shared our experiences of the day before. Some of the participants had not been able to experience the felt-shift, so Ed and Peter continued to work with them again that morning. Those of us who had successful Focusing experiences were told to break into pairs, one person being the facilitator leading the five step exercise, the other being the one guided.

Ed said that some people can go through the five-step Focusing process by themselves without anyone helping them, but he and Peter had found that it's easier to work with a Focusing companion.

That afternoon we had a surprise visitor. Dr. Eugene Gendlin, the grandfather of Focusing, had driven from Chicago to be with us in the workshop. An older guy with mussed up gray hair, he looked like the stereotypical college professor, but I felt I was in the presence of greatness. Here was someone who had advanced psychotherapy by helping people to learn the language of their own bodily knowing.

Dr. Gendlin talked to us for a few minutes about how pleased he was that Ed and Peter were advancing his Focusing concept into the spiritual dimension. He said he always believed the felt-shift was a gift one received in the

Focusing process. Peter and Ed called it grace, the state of being blessed and gifted by the favor of God. From my limited experience, I could certainly agree with them.

Focusing Spreads Throughout the World

Since that weekend in Wisconsin 24 years ago, Peter and Ed have gone on in their work with Focusing to accomplish some remarkable things. They have developed a non-profit organization called the Institute for BioSpiritual Research, located in the Denver area, from which to coordinate the many Focusing activities and resources available (see reference section). The office distributes a newsletter, and the secretary will answer any questions you may have about the Focusing movement. Books and video tapes are available to help people learn how to do Focusing, as well as information on Focusing seminars in various parts of the country There is a nominal yearly fee to become a member.

BioSpiritual Focusing groups have been formed in many parts of the country with the sole purpose of teaching people this valuable process of self-therapy. Meetings in the homes of friends and neighbors have helped thousands of people to facilitate each other in the Focusing process. Ed and Peter have shown me letters from people all over the country who report that by practicing Focusing, they have seen amazing changes for the better in their lives.

Ed and Peter have also set up BioSpiritual Focusing organizations internationally, in Mexico, Canada, England, Ireland and other countries. People in the Czech Republic have taken Focusing to the people in Bosnia, who sorely need psychological healing. I hope people in the Balkans who have experienced the healing-presence of BioSpiritual Focusing will take it to Kosovo to help those people deal with the extreme trauma of the murder, rape and other suffering they have experienced during the recent war.

I feel honored to have been the president of the Institute for BioSpiritual Research since its inception in 1975. Dolores and I and our family have helped the Institute financially through the years with funds from Caliana, our family foundation named after two very caring people, Dolores' mother Callie and my mother Anna. Peter Campbell and Ed McMahon have literally devoted their lives to spreading Focusing throughout the world. They, like Dr. Gendlin, will go down in history for their selfless contribution to the world's people who hunger for peace and happiness in their lives.

Try It Yourself!

You can try Focusing yourself by following the five steps as described in my workshop experience with Peter and Ed. If you need more help, I urge you to contact the national office of the Institute for BioSpiritual Research and see if you can learn the process through the books and tapes they offer. If you still don't get the hang of it, maybe you'll feel it's important enough in your life to fly or take the Amtrak to one of the Focusing Workshops listed in the literature available from the national office. Dolores and I flew to Wisconsin from Florida, because we thought it would make a difference in our lives, and it has. Or maybe you'll be lucky enough to find a workshop within driving distance. Whatever you do, I know you'll find it well worth the effort to bring Focusing into your life.

Chapter 8
Listen to the Spirit Within

In most Western religions, whether ours is the one we were born into or the one we currently profess, we learn that God is our father, and we are God's children. This is what I was taught growing up in the Catholic faith. But as a child, I became confused about my relationship with God. Even though I was taught that God loved me, I didn't really feel His love.

In my previous book, I wrote about a little pamphlet that changed my attitude toward God, entitled "Confidence in God," by Father Considine. Father Considine's thoughts about man's relationship to God as expressed in this little pamphlet were right on the mark for me:

> If we don't look upon God as a hard man, we have every reason to congratulate ourselves. We say we think Him merciful, kind, loving, but in our hearts we look upon Him as hard. Three-quarters of the troubles of good people come from this. He feels intensely our misconception of Him. We look upon Him as a hard,

grasping man, who wants to get all He can out of us and gives nothing in return. And woe betide us if we fail to satisfy Him. This is utterly wrong.

If God has ever shown me any love, He must love me still. God does not care for me one day and hate me the next. He is not capricious or inconstant like man. Above everything, God wants my love, and with love comes happiness and enthusiasm in His service. We think: I have one talent; others have five. Therefore, I will do nothing but bury mine. I will run no risks. But each of our temperaments and characters has been fitted exactly, thought out from all time, to suit our lives. What we have, we don't value; what we have not, we desire. Do not say that God, evidently, from my capabilities, does not care much for me, does not expect much from me. God craves our love. Ask, ask, ask for graces, and you will assuredly get them.

I didn't come across these words of Father Considine until I was married with a couple of children, but I was glad to have found his pamphlet because it started me on a path toward a loving relationship with God in my life.

In the pamphlet, Father Considine goes on to say:

Watch the present. Do not cry over spilt milk. Do not dwell on the faults and sins of the past. Leave them alone; leave them to God. Tell God you're sorry for those sins and never think of them again. Often the despondence caused by sin is more wrong and keeps one away from God more than sin itself. Don't waste time being discouraged. Get up and go to God. Draw near to Him. Do not stand back hanging your head.

He then says: "Do what thou doest." I interpret these words to mean that we should do what we are born to do in our lives. He continues:

> We need to look at the talents God gave us and use the temperaments and characters He gave us to decide what we want to do with our lives. Then we must think about it and work on it until we develop a passion to accomplish it. Only when we listen to the spirit within and do what God meant for us to be doing in our lives, will we really be happy.

It is through listening to the spirit within that we are guided on the path God intends for us—to "do what thou doest." Many call this an expression of God's will in our lives.

We need to think about what God's will is for us in our lives, because for each one of us it is different. We must look at the talent or talents God gave us, and how our "temperaments and characters have been fitted exactly, thought out from all time, to suit our lives," as Father Considine states so beautifully in his pamphlet.

Over the course of my life, I have tried to listen to the spirit within and to understand what God's will has been for me. Looking back, it seems I was guided on the path that God intended for me, and when I followed it, I was rewarded with happiness and success.

When I graduated from high school in 1940, I wanted to go to college to study accounting and business, but my dad couldn't afford to send me. My dad had been in business all of his life, and I admired him for this. He had owned a route of cigarette vending machines, and during my high school years, I helped him with the office work and went along on Saturdays with my brothers to service the machines. The year I graduated, he sold the business and encouraged me to take a job with the new owner, a man named Plous, whose office was in a neighboring city. In addition to the cigarette machines, Plous also owned candy and peanut vending machines which I serviced for him.

After working for Plous for a year, I discovered that I didn't like being tied down to an 8 to 5 job, five days a week. I couldn't see myself doing this for the rest of my life, so I decided to go into the peanut vending machine business where I believed I could earn more than the $75 a month salary Plous was giving me. On my own, I would be my own boss, living my life as I saw fit.

I had a problem, though. I was just 18 and had always been a shy kid. I knew I would be afraid to talk to the merchants about placing my peanut machines in their businesses, so I asked Chuck, who serviced the cigarette machines for Plous, to go into business with me. I figured he had the salesman's personality and gift of gab to get the machines placed. Then I told my dad my plan, and he agreed to finance Chuck and me in the business.

For the next 50 years, I had a passion for the vending business, and that passion continued as the business changed from peanut to gumball machines, then to vending machines with small toys in plastic capsules, which we placed in supermarkets.

After 50 years, I retired and turned the business over to one of our sons to run as a family business. To keep busy, I took some writing courses and I developed a passion for writing. Now, I feel fulfilled and am enjoying my retirement years immensely.

I repeat the words of Father Considine: "Only when we listen to the spirit within and do what God meant for us to be doing in our lives, will we really be happy."

And I might add that even if you haven't been listening to the spirit within up until now, it's never too late to start.

Easing the Pain of Worry

Father Considine's words tell us how to ease the pain of worry:

> Some people always have one eye on the past and the other on the future instead of both on the present. Don't waste time deploring the past and being apprehensive of the future. Grace will be given to meet each day the difficulties of that day. It is this incessant worrying over the past and the future that prevents concentration. Leave the future in God's hands.

In my life, I have often been challenged to leave the future in God's hands many times. Sometimes I think I'm a born worrier, because I've had such hard lessons in learning how to do this.

Many years ago, Dolores and I went on a trip with our two youngest children to the Grand Canyon. One morning, we were browsing in a souvenir shop with the children at the rim of the canyon, when we lost track of our youngest son, Jonathan, who was then ten years old. Dolores and I had gone our separate ways in the shop, each thinking Jonathan was with the other. When we came back together, neither of us knew where he was. We were devastated, both fearing he'd left the shop and wandered outside to the rim of the Canyon where there were no guardrails to protect him from falling over the edge.

Desperate to find him, we decided to go in different directions to increase our chances. Dolores and our other son, Peter, went one way, and I went the other. As I searched, I felt like I was carrying a rock in my stomach. It seemed like an hour, but was probably only half an hour, when, weak from worry, I gave up and rejoined Dolores.

She had found him! He had never left the store and must have escaped our notice. I hugged and kissed him, and thanked God we had found him. It had truly been one of the most agonizing experiences of my life.

Another incident occurred early in our married life, when Dolores became sick with worry because I hadn't returned home from one of my frequent car trips at the expected time. It was winter in Wisconsin, and a severe storm was raging. I didn't think she might be worried about me and didn't phone to tell her I would be late. But when I got home, she was extremely upset and burst into tears of relief and happiness that I was safe.

I'm sure most of us have experienced this kind of intense and prolonged worry over some incident in our lives and would agree that it can be one of the most painful experiences a person can go through.

Tom, a jokester friend of mine, told me his solution for worry: "Write down your worries on a piece of paper," he advised, "and put the paper in an envelope with a ten dollar bill. Mail it to this little old lady who lives in Tennessee and sits in her rocking chair on her front porch opening the letters she gets from people all over the country. As she reads each one, she worries as she rocks, day in and day out, for all the people who have sent her their money!"

I chuckled at that one and thought about how foolish we are to worry so much in our daily lives. I would guess that 95% of the things I worry about never even happen.

I'd like to suggest another way to alleviate the pain of worry, and it won't cost you a single dime. Simply turn your worries over to God! So much of our worrying is usually over things we can't do anything about anyway, so why not let God worry for us?

It sounds easy, yet it's very difficult to do, unless we have already developed a deep trust and faith in God's love for us. I suggest we read over and over again the words of Father Considine as I have quoted him, to build our confidence in God and become thoroughly convinced that God loves us dearly and only wants good for us. Then we can ask God to shoulder our worries and have confidence that they will be among the 95% of those that never materialize.

While this works well for me, I can't say that I am completely relieved of my agonizing when I turn my worries over to God. But it is comforting to know God loves me and is sharing my worry, and that He has the power to protect me and prevent whatever it is I'm worried about from actually happening.

If I weren't able to put things in God's hands and be confident that He will protect me, I couldn't leave the house in the morning and drive down the road without worrying I might be in an accident. Have you ever thought of how God protects us when we're driving for hours on two-lane highways at 60 miles per hour with cars coming at us just as fast and passing with only a few feet between? And then there are the stupid things we do, such as not looking carefully enough before making a turn and having a near miss with another driver, barely avoiding an accident. When this happens to me, I always say out loud, "Thanks, God!"

In my years of business, I've had my share of financial worries, many of which I wrote about in my previous book. At times, my worrying caused me to experience chest pains so severe, I felt like a spike was being driven into my chest right through to my back. Twice, I went to the hospital and each time told the doctor I thought the pain was from worrying about my business. He felt it was best to check it anyway and had MRIs done on me that showed no damage had occurred anywhere in my body.

During those difficult times when I worried a lot about my business, I was able to get some relief by praying to God for help in carrying my burden. As a result, many times, my worries were seldom so severe as to disturb my sleep at night.

Even as recently as a few days ago, several small incidents happened that caused me to worry. One evening, a disturbing phone message was left on the answering machine, and I wasn't able to return the call until the next morning. When I did, I found there was nothing to be worried about; in fact, the situation had a pleasant outcome instead of the one I feared. In another incident, I was having trouble transmitting a manuscript to my editor on the computer, which gnawed at me for hours. Then a thought came to me: "If I turn my big worries over to God, why not the small ones, too?"

I realized that during most of my life, and especially

in my business, I had been constantly plagued with these kinds of petty, low-grade worries, and I had learned to live with them. My worrying even led me to making decisions I later regretted. Dolores tells me we could have made a lot of money in the stock market if I'd only listened to her when she urged me dozens of times to stop moving money around so often—sometimes monthly, even weekly—all because I was worried that my stock would go down.

So two days ago, I made a vow to myself to turn even my low-grade worries over to God. Why not, I asked myself, figuring that the small ones are certainly easier for God to handle than the big ones. And to make sure I wouldn't keep taking my worries back from God, I vowed that any time I found myself thinking about worrisome things, I would use the relaxation exercise (explained in another chapter of this book) to get my mind off my problems—no matter how big or how small. If I can only get the courage to include worrying about the stock market, think of all the money I might make!

A Personal Relationship with God

Many religions teach that God dwells within us. If this is true, and God is not some remote power we have little access to, wouldn't it be wonderful to experience having a personal relationship with Him in our lives?

As a Catholic with a strong desire for a more personal relationship with God, I'm disappointed I don't hear very much about this concept in our Catholic churches. As I've told my priest friends, I hear more about having a personal relationship with God on the TV services of various charismatic denominations than I do on Sunday morning in our Catholic churches.

I first heard about having a personal relationship with God when Dolores and I joined a Protestant charismatic group, and then later a group of Catholic charismatics, for what they call prayer meetings. It was at these weekly meetings that I came to understand what it meant to have a personal relationship with God. I was fascinated when people stood up and "witnessed," or spoke about how God had been active in their personal lives during the previous week. Some talked about how their prayers had been answered and how this had increased their faith. Others told about the small miracles that occurred when they or family members changed their ways for the better as a result of talking personally to God.

Over the years, my relationship with God has changed from the time I was a confused child and didn't feel that God loved me. I have developed faith and now know that God loves Dolores and me, and our children, and only wants good things for us. I personally ask God to help us all love and care for each other, and to do the same for others who enter our lives. I feel we are all making progress, and this is demonstrated in both our business and family life.

Several years ago, Dolores and I gifted our gumball and toy vending machine business to our eight children. One of them took over the management of the business six years ago when I retired, and is doing a great job as president of the company. We have now held two family shareholder meetings, one this year and one a year ago.

At the first meeting, we needed to get agreement from all the children about how much compensation and stock ownership the president should receive. This took a lot of negotiation, and things did not go smoothly. But at this year's meeting, helped by a lot of prayers to God, we have come to a reasonable settlement that I believe all can live with. The love and affection the children now show for Dolores and me, and for each other, seemed unattainable only a year ago.

However, I am a firm believer that prayer alone doesn't solve problems. In order to resolve the conflicts that arose a year ago in our family, we all had to learn to work together, each sharing and accepting the others' ideas. Besides asking God for help, we had to put in the hard work of getting along with each other.

For me, having a personal relationship with God has come to mean talking with God in the quiet of my mind, which I believe is prayer, and sometimes getting answers about what I should or shouldn't do through my intuition. This personal relationship also includes feeling the protection of God that I mentioned earlier.

My relationship with God has become very important to me in my writing. When I sit down to write, I take some time, usually 10 or 15 minutes, to do my relaxation exercise and clear my mind of all the things that are bombarding it. Then I ask God to help me with my writing by assembling a team of people who have passed on: our son John, who died shortly after birth; my parents and brothers and sisters, especially Joseph and Louise whom I've never met since they died before I was born; Dolores' family members; my army buddy Tony Wilhelm, a good friend and a very successful writer; Mother Theresa (I always ask if she has the time to help me, of course!) and Saint Francis Xavier, the patron saint of writers. Thanks to all this help, I haven't experienced writer's block once in the many years I've been writing.

What It Means to Have Free Will

Most religions acknowledge that God has given us all the free will to accept or reject Him in our lives. In other words, it's entirely up to us. God didn't make us all robots, unable to choose freely, but instead gave us the free will to love or not love Him, as well as our fellow man, to get close or stay our distance. But I also believe God dearly wants us to love Him and to share His love with each other.

Sometimes our free will takes us away from God. But I don't believe God punishes people because God doesn't operate that way. God is the epitome of goodness. As parents, we realize that our children also have a free will. Sometimes we see them stray from our teaching, and we punish them in order to make them change their ways.

While I don't think God punishes us, I do think He allows us to experience what we may perceive as punishment in the form of illness and natural disasters. Man's own free will however, is responsible for other adversities in our lives—war, death camps, murder, accidents, and the hurts and problems we cause each other.

I believe God's main goal for us during our lives here on earth is our spiritual salvation, and any way this can be accomplished is fair game to Him. Therefore, He allows disasters to happen in our lives as a way of bringing us to spiritual salvation. We have all heard stories about soldiers on the battlefield getting converted when, lost and helpless in their final hour, they turned to God as a last resort. Similarly, I think God allows repeated adversity in our daily lives so we can experience conversion after conversion and are brought closer to that ultimate goal which I think is supernatural life here on earth.

I believe God answers all prayers, even when He seems to not answer them. By doing nothing in response to some of our prayers, He may well be acting in our best interest.

What is God's will for us in this life? That's for each of us to find — how best to accomplish our spiritual salvation, or, as some might say, how to "get to Heaven."

I believe we are all here for a purpose, and that maybe for some of us, that purpose is to help others to get to Heaven. By doing so, we eventually get there ourselves.

If things don't seem to be going right in our lives, maybe we need to look into ourselves to see if something we are doing, thinking, or saying is blocking us from knowing what God's will is for us. Sometimes God's will isn't our will, and this can cause quite a conflict of interests. It's truly wonderful when our will coincides with God's, because then our lives become much easier and eventually much happier.

A Deep Gratitude

For some people, getting to Heaven is something they accomplish while still here on earth. In other words, they find Heaven on earth. I believe I might be one of those fortunate people, and I feel deep gratitude for all I have been given.

Daily, I thank God for a wonderful, loving wife and for eight wonderful, loving children. I thank God for two beautiful homes in beautiful settings, one in Door County, Wisconsin, where temperatures range from 60-80 degrees in the summers, and the other in Santa Barbara, California, where for the balance of the year, the climate is equally as pleasant. I thank God that all of our children are making a living for themselves and their families, and that our family business supplies enough so Dolores and I and our children, and possibly even our grandchildren, should never have to face the hard times Dolores and I did as children during the Depression years. I thank God that they are all good kids and are close to God and to each other. I thank God for the wonderful friends we have in both the locations in which we live and for our good health, and that of our children and grandchildren. I thank God for our business that was often fun for me to run, and that one of our children seems to be even better at running than I was. I thank God I've found a new career in writing which I can thoroughly enjoy in my retirement. And finally, I thank God that I can pass on to others some of the things I have learned in my life to make their lives a bit more healthy and happy.

REFERENCES & RESOURCES

Diana Schwarzbein, MD
"So it May Be True After All:Eating Pasta Makes You Fat."- NY Times,1995
"New Skinny on Low-fat Diet Trend." - Santa Barbara News Press, 1995

        Recommended:
        "The Schwarzbein Principle" with Nancy Deville;
        "The Schwarzbein Principle Cookbook" and
        "The Schwarzbein Principle Vegetarian Cookbook" with
            Nancy Deville and Evelyn Jacob Jaffee

        All published by:
        Health Communications, Inc.
        3201 SW 15th St
        Dearfield Beach, FL   33442-8190

Barry Sears, Ph.D.
"The Zone" Harper Collins Inc., New York, NY, 1996

Candace Pert, Ph.D.
"The Molecules of Emotion" Scribners, New York, NY, 1997

Corinne T. Netzer
"The Complete Book of Food Counts"
        Dell Readers Service
        Box DR, 1540 Broadway
        New York, NY 10036

Maxwell Maltz, MD
"Psycho-Cybernetics"
        Out of Print
        Simon & Schuster, Inc.
        New York, NY, 1960

Books and Tapes on *Focusing*

Eugene Gendlin, Ph.D.
"Focusing" Everest House, New York, NY. 1978

Edwin McMahon, Ph.D.
"Beyond the Myth of Dominance"
        Book Masters, Inc.
        PO Box 388
        Mansfield, OH 44805
        Ph. 800-247-6553

Peter Campbell, Ph.D. &
Edwin McMahon, Ph.D.
"BioSpirituality: Focusing as a Way to Grow"
        Loyola Press
        3441 N. Ashland Ave.
        Chicago, IL 60657
        Ph. 800-621-1008
        Online: http://www.amazon.com

BioSpirituality Focusing Videotapes

Nada Lou Productions
908 Lake St. Louis Road
Ville de Lery, Quebec
Canada J6N 1A7
Ph/F: 450-692-9339

BioSpiritual Focusing National Headquarters

Institute for BioSpiritual Research
PO Box 741137
Arvada, CO 80006-1137
Ph/F:303-427-5311
e-mail: LFLOM@mho.net

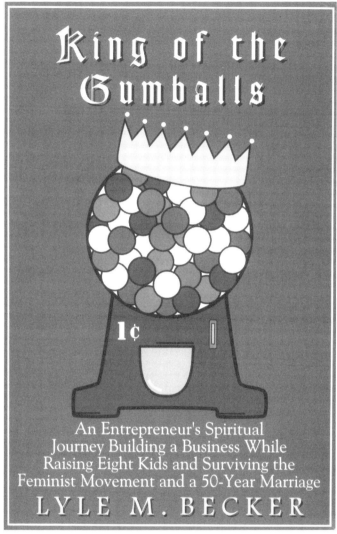

King of the
Gumballs

1¢

An Entrepreneur's Spiritual
Journey Building a Business While
Raising Eight Kids and Surviving the
Feminist Movement and a 50-Year Marriage
LYLE M. BECKER

ABOUT THE AUTHOR

Lyle Becker began writing six years ago as a second career after retiring at 72 after 52 years in the vending machine business, turning the business over to his son to run. An entrepreneur at 18, one year out of high school, he started in the vending business with 300 peanut machines and built a successful national business of toy and bubble gum machines in supermarkets throughout the country. His first book *King of the Gumballs*, tells the story of how he struggled to build the business while his wife, Dolores, almost single-handedly raised their eight children. Now, feeling like he's in his fifties, he shares what he has learned these past 76 years listening to his body and, God willing, adding many happy healthy years to his life span. He tells you how you can do the same. He writes from their homes on Moonlight Bay in Door County, Wisconsin and in Santa Barbara, California.